Understanding Plague

Studies in the Humanities
Literature—Politics—Society

Guy Mermier
General Editor

Vol. 68

PETER LANG
New York • Washington, D.C./Baltimore • Bern
Frankfurt am Main • Berlin • Brussels • Vienna • Oxford

Randal P. Garza

Understanding Plague

The Medical and Imaginative Texts of Medieval Spain

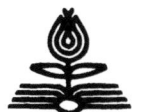

PETER LANG
New York • Washington, D.C./Baltimore • Bern
Frankfurt am Main • Berlin • Brussels • Vienna • Oxford

Library of Congress Cataloging-in-Publication Data

Garza, Randal Paul.
Understanding plague: the medical and imaginative texts
of medieval Spain / Randal P. Garza.
p. cm. — (Studies in the humanities; v. 68)
Originally presented as the author's thesis (Ph.D.)—
Michigan State University.
Dept. of Romance and Classical Languages, 2001.
Includes bibliographical references.
1. Plague—Spain—History—15th century. 2. Medicine,
Medieval—Spain. 3. Medicine—Historiography.
[DNLM: 1. Plague—history—Spain. 2. Disease Outbreaks—history—Spain.
3. History, 15th Century—Spain. 4. History, Medieval—Spain.
5. Medicine in Literature—Spain. WC 350 G245u 2008] I. Title.
II. Studies in the humanities (New York, N.Y.); v. 68.
RC178.S7G37   616.9′232—dc22   2007041547
ISBN 978-0-8204-6341-4
ISSN 0742-6712

Bibliographic information published by **Die Deutsche Bibliothek**.
Die Deutsche Bibliothek lists this publication in the "Deutsche
Nationalbibliografie"; detailed bibliographic data is available
on the Internet at http://dnb.ddb.de/.

© 2008 Peter Lang Publishing, Inc., New York
29 Broadway, 18th floor, New York, NY 10006
www.peterlang.com

All rights reserved.
Reprint or reproduction, even partially, in all forms such as microfilm,
xerography, microfiche, microcard, and offset strictly prohibited.

Table of Contents

Acknowledgments vii

Introduction 1

CHAPTER ONE
Historical Interpretations of Plague 13
    Mimêsis and Early Historical Plague Writing........................... 14

CHAPTER TWO
Medical Writing / Treatises of Medieval Spain 29
    "Del regimiento en tienpo de pestilencia," *Menor daño de medicina*. Segunda parte del regimiento de sanidat, Capítulo XIII. Alonso de Chirino 42
    "Tratado útil y muy provechoso contra toda pestilencia y aire corupto." Licenciado Fores.. 47

CHAPTER THREE
Allusions to Plague: Themes in the Fictional Texts
    of the Iberian Peninsula 57
    Libro de (la) miseria d'omne 71
    Revelaçión de un hermitanno... 78
    La dança general de la Muerte 85

Conclusion 101

Bibliography 115

Acknowledgments

The publication of this book was made possible thanks to the generosity of the University of Tennessee at Martin Office of Research, Grants and Contracts, the College of Humanities and Fine Arts and the Department of Modern Foreign Languages.

Introduction

This study has come about owing to my interest in examining how the threat of widespread contagious disease could have affected the society in which it occurred. It is, therefore, an investigation of Spanish medical and literary works that share the common trait of being produced around the years of virulent plague epidemics in the Iberian Peninsula. In bringing together for comparison and analysis diverse works produced from the late 14th to the mid 16th centuries, a period marking the shift from the late Middle to Early Modern Spain, this investigation hopes to aid in filling a void that has long gone unnoticed by critics worldwide. In his 1969 publication, *The Black Death*, Philip Ziegler makes a comment that—unfortunately—still holds true today: "no major study of the Black Death in the Iberian Peninsula has yet been written" (85). Indeed, this void is striking when compared with intellectual activity in other European countries such as England, France and Germany—all of which have produced a vast array of primary and secondary information with regard to plague and especially the Black Death of 1348. Critical attention to and assessment of the social and literary impact of the Black Death in Spain has been, by contrast, conspicuously limited. One readily apparent explanation for this deficiency is our lack of precise historical information and direct references in imaginative texts that address the issue of plague in Spain. In comparison with other nations which possess a far richer body of texts documenting both the demographic as well as the psychological devastation of medieval plague, similar resources dealing with the Iberian Peninsula are relatively scarce. This is especially true when it comes to its literature. While other western cultures have major fictional works produced around the time of lethal outbreaks that directly comment on the plague,[1] the small number of literary texts produced near the outbreaks of plague in Spain is not as copious in its direct references to plague. It is precisely the absences, the silences and the ambiguities regarding these medieval Spanish texts at the time of plague that aroused interest and gave rise to this study.

Currently, modern research generally concedes that the pernicious disease that ravaged most of medieval Europe was a human tragedy with a widespread and profound impact on economic and social behavior. However, this present state of scholarly opinion has not always been the case. Plague research over the years has experienced a marked evolution of theories in which the views of one generation of critics are quickly debunked and replaced by subsequent counter reactions. This holds true for the critical opinion concerning the plague both in Spain and in Europe as a whole. As a result, plague criticism over the years has produced a broad spectrum of conclusions that often contradict one another in their attempt to establish even the most basic elements of plague history. Thus, we find frequent disputes among critics in what pertains to the years involving major plague epidemics as well as the consequential mortality rates.[2]

The dominant critical view which was prevalent from the around the mid-nineteenth to the beginning of the twentieth century, characterized the widespread socio-economic changes marking the end of the Middle Ages and the beginning of the Renaissance as caused by the lethal plague pandemic popularly referred to as the Black Death.[3] Reaching maximum virulence in Western Europe c. 1348, this well known biological disaster was typically regarded by early researchers to be epochal in nature due to the incredibly high estimated mortality rates associated with the outbreak. One early critic who espoused this perception was J.F.C. Hecker who concludes in a study published in 1846 that the Black Death alone was "one of the most important events which have prepared the way for the present state of Europe" (31). Taking this conclusion even further, A.L. Maycock also agrees that "the year 1348 marks the nearest approach to a definite break in the continuity of history that has ever occurred" (quoted in Campbell, 4). Similar to the way in which modern geologists consider the impact of a giant comet or asteroid to be the catastrophic event marking the boundary between Cretaceous and Tertiary periods, early plague researchers estimated the mortality caused by the Black Death to be so high that the event could have had nothing but disastrous consequences. Clearly, with some early researchers overestimating mortality rates of the Black Death to as much as nine tenths of the total population of Europe, the natural conclusions to be drawn from such a high figure would portray the event as catastrophic to society. However, because they were faced with a fundamental lack of reliable demographic evidence with which to accurately gauge mortality rates, early researchers of medieval plague were forced to develop various models in order to extrapolate their figures. It is precisely the inevitable questioning of these initial figures that eventually inspired an equally strong moderating counter reaction to those early estimates.

Beginning around the 1920s, plague criticism evolved in a direction that was openly skeptical of the conclusions of previous researchers. At a time when logical positivism was at the philosophical forefront of many academic disciplines, the importance of scientific verification of data was paramount to the acquisition of knowledge: as in other fields, there were new advances made in the field of plague investigation. While earlier historians had placed the estimated mortality rate as high as nine-tenths of the population, backed by positivist methods of research, a new generation of scholars set the death rate as low as twenty-five percent—a percentage obviously too low to have provoked any widespread change. One scholar, Anna M. Campbell, began by suggesting that the conclusions made by earlier researchers of medieval plague came to be so exaggerated due to their unquestioning acceptance of first-hand accounts as solid fact. Thus, the exaggerated figures and conclusions of the early researchers were seen as reflecting the emotional impression of the medieval chroniclers who tended to overstate the devastation caused by the epidemic around them. Campbell explains that late-nineteenth to early-twentieth century historians typically estimated mortality rates at three-fourths and two-thirds of the population. This view also directly correlates with the contemporary chroniclers of plague—such as the papal physicians, Guy of Chauliac and Chalin of Vivario—who tried to accurately document the widespread damage that surrounded them. Showing, in all probabilities, the influence of their own personal fears, Campbell notes that these chroniclers "more often approach the higher figure, frequently exceeding it" (2). Recognizing this propensity for exaggeration, the new breed of 1920 plague scholars—armed with new theoretical models of academic research such as positivism—began to debunk the highest mortality estimates as having been inaccurately influenced by emotion.[4] It was their opinion that the initial evidence compiled from religious, university and hospital records that made specific reference to plague and the Black Death, was insufficient to support such high death estimates. Ultimately, this thought led to a marked decrease of critical opinion concerning the impact and importance of medieval plague in general.

Finally, modern results of medieval plague study have come full circle and, in so doing, they have established a more comprehensive approach that serves as the foundation of this study. Questioning the extremely high as well as unrealistically low mortality rates attributed to the Black Death, authors such as David Herlihy saw the Black Death in Europe as only one isolated episode in a larger series of plague epidemics. In 1958, Herlihy published a study that not only reaffirms the exceptionally high mortality rates of the plague pandemic in Europe, setting the figure as high as seventy to eighty percent of the population of some villages, but he also offers an expanded scope for approaching plague studies.

One of Herlihy's most interesting conclusions was that: "The Black Death of 1348 and 1349, and *the recurrent epidemics of the fourteenth and fifteenth centuries* [emphasis added], were the most devastating natural disasters ever to strike Europe" (16). In Herlihy's opinion, it is the recurrent nature of plague, and not just the Black Death of 1348–1349, that was to blame for the catastrophic losses in population. In short, once the Black Death exacted its high toll of human life, subsequent plague outbreaks continued to hold population levels in check and it is this extended check on population levels that effected the most sweeping changes at both the demographic and psychological levels. Randolph Starn is in complete agreement with Herlihy and, commenting on a terrible plague that ravaged Italy in 1630–31, summarizes the current trends in plague research in these terms:

> Twenty years ago, Bartolomé Bennassar outlined a research agenda divided into topics and subtopics and ranging from the medical, demographic, and economic to the social and religious aspects of the "great epidemics" of the Mediterranean world. The latest bibliographies list dozens of studies on these subjects.[5] As a result of these investigations, much more is known

about general patterns as well as specific details, and this knowledge has begun to transform some long-standing assumptions. On the graphs of historical demographers and economic historians, which extend over generations and even centuries, recurrent epidemics are likely to appear less the exception than the rule, all the more so when "lesser plagues" are identified in the company of the greater ones or in the intervals between them: sickness rather than health thus becomes the "normal" human condition. (quoted in Calvi, "Introduction": x)

This rather more chronic nature of plague, therefore, is currently defining the search for and identification of medieval society's response to the constant threat of lethal epidemics. In terms of demographics and historical reactions, this task is relatively straightforward as institutional responses such as public health regulations and death records are easily quantifiable. However, following in the footsteps of Bennassar, modern research strives for something more: a desire to understand plague at the human level as the experience of living with a recurrent biological threat would necessarily affect human feelings, behavior and imagination. As world literature produced during and immediately following periods of plague virulence affords the greatest insight into human reactions to the calamity, textual analysis and the resulting themes identified is the current focus of modern research. In that which concerns medieval Spain since the onset of the Black Death, this is also another specific interest of this study.

In the chapters that follow, we will bring together for comparison and analysis a number of medieval works of both historical and literary nature produced in the Iberian Peninsula in the years surrounding virulent plague epidemics. In order to establish the timeframe from which we may justify our selection of examples, it will first be useful to review the periods that modern researchers currently associate with the greatest plague outbreaks in medieval Spain.

In 1956, Amada López de Meneses published a rich source of 157 historical documents that make specific mention of the Black Death in Aragon spanning the years 1348 to 1384. Beginning with a letter of Pedro IV in April, 1348 that discusses possible steps to deter the coming of plague, until final entry of Prince Don Juan which still openly shows fear of contagion as late as May 1384, this body of documents does much to establish the initial timeframe and dramatic consequences of this major pandemic in Spain.⁶

Clearly, as subsequent studies based on the original documents of López de Meneses demonstrate, the same level of disruption and disorder that characterized the effects of the disease in the rest of Europe affected the major port cities of the Iberian Peninsula in a quite similar fashion. In 1973, Jaime Sobrequés Callicó produced a detailed historiographical account in which he traces the effects of the Black Death in a region-by-region study of the Iberian Peninsula. Based in part on the study of López de Meneses, Sobrequés Callicó's primary conclusions were that the pandemic that reached the Peninsula in 1348, affecting society at the social, economic and political levels, also reoccurred with similar virulence in both 1362 and 1384. Alan Deyermond confirms this phenomenon by noting the cyclical nature of plague in the Iberian Peninsula: "The Black Death (pneumonic and bubonic plague) first struck Spain in 1348, with further epidemics in 1362 and the 1370s" (*The Middle Ages*, 118). Despite the obvious discrepancy with regard to the specific years of major plague outbreaks, both Sobrequés Callicó and Deyermond touch upon an important and currently undisputed fact: the deadly plague outbreak of c.1348—so well documented in literary studies—was not an isolated event but rather one in a series of lethal epidemics.

In 1988, Marcelino Amasuno presented a wider panorama of the onset and course of plague in medieval Spain and came to the conclusion that the historical phenomenon that detonated widespread changes at all levels of European life had equally significant consequences in the Iberian Peninsula.⁷ In spite of the resistance of earlier scholars to accept that the pernicious disease that played havoc with much of the world also affected Spain to a similar degree, Amasuno used references to plague in historical documents to compile a more detailed and complete chronology of the epidemic. His conclusion was that traditional scholars had been too conservative in their assumption that plague in the Iberian Peninsula reached only Portugal, Galicia and Castile. Indeed, that widespread disease affected a far greater number of Iberian cities and towns in the same cyclical patterns that had been documented throughout the rest of Europe. At the time of the Black Death, plague reached Barcelona and Valencia in May of 1348 and continued its journey southward to Almería in June of that same year. Uncharacteristically remaining active throughout the autumn and winter, this first viral wave is known to have lasted at least until March of 1350 when it killed Alfonso XI, the king of Castile.[8] However, according to Amasuno, the true *long-term* effects of plague in the Iberian Peninsula were not due to the Black Death—one single plague outbreak. It is more accurate to recognize that the epidemiological phenomenon in Iberia mirrors what we know happened in the rest of the world and reoccurred with frequency in the years to come. By closely analyzing documents produced during the time of plague outbreaks subsequent to 1348–1349, Amasuno concludes:

> Así pues, puede decirse que se abre el siglo XV con una epidemia pestosa que posiblemente alcanzará una considerable incidencia en el reino de Castilla y que anticipa, en su primer tercio, cuatro importantes brotes pestíferos que se sitúan en los siguientes períodos cronológicos: 1413–1414, 1422, 1426–1427, 1429 y 1431. (Medicina castellano-leonesa, 11).

Frequently recurring with brutal intensity and spanning nearly one hundred years from start to finish, this pestilential disease would have clearly influenced life and letters in the Iberian Peninsula.

With current historiographic evidence now leading modern researchers to conclude that the recurring plagues that ravaged the rest of Europe also attacked medieval Spain with equally high mortality rates, the question turns to how this extended calamity affected the society in which it occurred. It is well-known that both purely fictional as well as old historical writing—itself, in part, a product of the imagination—has been drawn to the topic of plague since antiquity. It was through the expressive form of writing that early authors such as Thucydides and Procopius sought to make sense out of the chaos and disorder that accompanied the pestilential outbreaks of their respective times. In the eyes of plague scholars such as Barbara Fass Leavy, René Girard and David Steel, it is this goal of using the written word as a means of comprehending a misunderstood biological calamity that unites all forms of plague writing. Despite the chronological distance that separates one work of plague literature from the next, writings from the Bible to the modern accounts of AIDS, Ebola and the Hanta virus, then, all share a remarkably similar "standard" version of portraying the visitation: "A historical actor (the leader, the city, the Christian people, the nation) receives from an outside source (God, foreign lands, the Jews, social deviants) an infection (punishment, test) for which the actor must seek the proper remedy (prayer, science, exile, extermination)."[9] By bringing together several works of medieval Spanish literature for comparison and analysis, it will become clear that there were, indeed, marked changes in the portrayal of death in and around the greatest years of plague mortality. What we will see is a movement towards a more realistic and morbidly graphic portrayal of death and dying. Reflecting a changing philosophy of the meaning of both death and life, this new imagery will concentrate, above all, on Huizinga's idea of the putrefying corpse: "the concrete embodiment of the perishable."[10]

Accurate mortality rates do not matter as much when treating of the cultural impact of plague as a pandemic necessarily affects the lives of everyone around it. Lethal epidemic events of a widespread and cyclical nature affect every member—whether infected or not—of a society. It is human nature for those afflicted with a deadly infection to question despairingly their actions in an attempt to discover an explanation for their death sentence.

In the Middle Ages, changing societal perceptions towards the figures of Life and Death has been previously championed by critics such as Huizinga and Tristram. In his detailed study of English literature, *Figures of Life and Death in Medieval English Literature*, Tristram even goes so far as to conclude that the Western figures of Life and Death which are considered commonplace today were originally developed (though not invented) in the period 1350–1500s.[11] For Tristram, this evolution of images occurred for a reason:

> Because the medieval spectrum of beliefs about life and death was so much wider than ours, it reached to greater extremes: the strenuous vision, on the one hand, of eternal beatitude, led, on the other to the desolation of wan hope, the despair of those many who could no longer, with confidence, affirm their expectation of immortality. Just as the meaningless cycle of mutability came, at the end of the Middle Ages, to dominate the more purposeful rhythms of nature and transience, so morbid imaginings of the detail of decay displaced the affirmation of resurrection. (152)

The proliferation of dark images representing physical corruption in such a detailed manner sought to shock its audience through an attack on the senses. In this respect, literary works of the time abound with descriptions that attempt to both repulse at the visual level with the macabre representation of corporal decay—as well as to repel at the olfactory level—with graphic elaboration of the putrid odors that accompany physical decomposition. Never before had the image of human beauty turning to decay been depicted in such graphically realistic terms. But this new phenomenon did not occur arbitrarily in time: this new macabre interest in representing death and decay corresponds precisely with the documented years of plague epidemics and is directly correlated with prevailing views of the faithful concerning this life and the afterlife.

Obviously, as with any calamity of such large proportions, the reaction of the individual members of a society in which it occurs is not uniform. Robert E. Lerner illustrates the point with this graphic account:

> Robert Benchley once remarked that in every news photo of epoch-making events there always seems to be a man in a derby hat looking in the opposite direction from the action: on Bloody Sunday in St. Petersburg or assassination day in Sarajevo, a 'Johnny-on-the-spot' is always looking up at a clock, picking his teeth, or waving insouciantly at the camera. (77–78)

This perfectly understandable individual reaction to a calamity has never been more evident than in medieval Spain where the mountainous topography would undoubtedly keep entire villages out of harm's way. Citizens of such a region most likely would not have been thrust into the center of a storm, brought face-to-face with thoughts about the end of the world or their spiritual place in the universe. Likewise, it is conceivable that many who actually were faced with the reality of lethal contagion might not have accepted the disease as an eschatological warning, signaling the end of the world. However, it is indisputable that this widespread calamity would have led many to consider the disease a punitive visitation from God and, as such, wonder how the calamity fit into His plans. The consideration of possible answers to this question by contemporaries of the period is precisely our interest here.

While modern studies continue to find new literary and artistic evidence in support of the changing medieval philosophy concerning faith and the afterlife in western countries such as England, France and Germany, to date no such study has been carried out for Spanish literature. To assist in filling that void, this study brings together for comparison and analysis several works of medieval Spanish literature that all were produced during or immediately after plague epidemics and, in their subject matter, all show the strong influence of the calamitous period in which its author lived. Admittedly, it is certain that plague cannot have been the sole inspiration of the works presented here. However, it is also inconceivable that plague pandemics that exacted regularly high mortality rates from every strata of society would not have affected the historical and literary production of writers of that era. What we shall place on display here is the proof that literary works invoking the morbid and realistic depictions of physical decay and corruption that evolve from around the 1350s to the 1500s in other European countries also occur in the literature of Spain at this same time. As we shall demonstrate, the time period chosen is not an arbitrary one; rather, it correlates directly with the results of modern research on plague epidemics in medieval Iberia. Thus, as this is in no way an attempt to write a comprehensive history of the changing representations of death and dying in medieval Spain, we will use the historical dates associated with plague outbreaks—specifically, the years 1348–1349, 1362–1370, 1384, 1413–1414, 1422, 1426–1427, 1429 and 1431—as the criterion by which to justify the selection of texts.

Notes

1. Such works would include Giovanni Boccaccio's *The Decameron* or Geoffrey Chaucer's *The Pardoner's Tale*.
2. In 1985, Julio Valdeón reaffirms the difficulty of tracing the evolution and quantifying the impact of the Black Death in the Iberian Peninsula. While he begins by affirming that there is no doubt that the Black Death was the greatest single event to negatively impact the Iberian Peninsula of the fourteenth century, he also admits that: "No es fácil reconstruir ni la cronología ni el itinerario seguidos por la Peste Negra en su propagación por la Península Ibérica (...). Cuantificar la mortandad causada por la Peste Negra es de todo punto imposible, salvo, a lo sumo, para determinados ámbitos regionales o locales" (19–22).
3. It should be noted that terminology here is especially important as this study makes deliberate distinctions between the Black Death—referring to the specific outbreak of the mid–fourteenth century—and medieval plague—the recurrent epidemic phenomenon. Rosemary Horrox makes this similar distinction: "The name 'Black Death' is a later coinage. Contemporaries do not seem to have put a name to the illness, referring to it in non-specific ways as a mortality or epidemic. Even the words plague or pestilence, which became the standard terms for the disease, were originally non-specific, and have remained so: not all plagues are *the* plague" (3–4). In this sense, the Black Death is considered one specific biological event in the larger pattern of chronic pestilent disease in the Middle Ages.
4. Charles Verlinden, a former professor at the University of Gand and director of the Academia Belgica in Rome, authored a well-known study in 1938 that also presents an ultra-conservative opinion of the Black Death and its effects on Spain. While openly admitting that it is impossible to give any sort of "controllable statistics" for suffering directly caused by plague, he concludes that the great plague did, in fact, have little overall social or political impact on Spain or Europe as a whole. (from "La Grande Pest de 1348 en Espagne," *Revue Belge de Philologie et d'Histoire*, 17 (1938), 143–146, translated by William M. Bowsky).
5. See Bartolomé Bennassar, *Recherches sur les grandes épidémies dans le Nord de l'Espagne à la fin du XIVe siècle* (Paris: PU du Mirail, 1969); and the bibliographical essay by Ann G. Carmichael, *Plague and the Poor in Renaissance Florence* (New York: Cambridge UP, 1986): 166–75.
6. For a detailed study and interpretation of the documents published by López de Meneses, see Melanie V. Shirk, "The Black Death in Aragon, 1348–1351," *Journal of Medieval History*, 7 (1981): 357–367.

7. See Marcelino V. Amasuno, *Contribución al estudio del fenómeno epidémico en la Castilla de la primera mitad del siglo XV: el <<Regimiento contra la Pestilencia>> de Alfonso López de Valladolid*, (Valladolid: U de Valladolid, 1998).
8. Philip Ziegler notes that although the plague affected the royal house of Aragon by killing King Pedro's youngest daughter and niece in May and his wife in October, the detrimental consequences were far greater to the kingdom of Castile:

> The disease spread next through Arab Spain so that the armies confronting Alfonso XI were afflicted before their Christian enemies. It is said that the Arabs were deeply disturbed by this phenomenon and many of them seriously thought of adopting Christianity as a form of preventative medicine. Fortunately for their faith, however, the Black Death was soon raging quite as disastrously among the troops of Castile (…). The Castilian army in front of Gibraltar survived inviolate through 1349; then, in March, 1350, was suddenly attacked by the plague. The senior officers begged King Alfonso to leave his troops and seek safety in isolation but he refused to do so. He duly caught the disease and died on Good Friday, 26 March, 1350. He was the only ruling monarch of Europe to perish during the Black Death" (86).

9. Jean-Pierre Peter and Jacques Revel, "Le corps: L'homme malade et son histoire," as translated by Randolph Starn, forward to G. Calvi, x.
10. Taken from Johan Huizinga, *The Waning of the Middle Ages, 138.*
11. See Phillipa Tristram, *The Figures of Life and Death in Medieval English Literature*, 1.

• CHAPTER ONE •

Historical Interpretations of Plague

> Ever since the wails from the Philistine cities rose to heaven, plague has regularly marred the history of civilization, most often as isolated outbreaks affecting only a single city or a small region. Three times, however, vast plague pandemics have ravished nearly the whole of the inhabited world. (Gregg, 4)

From the earliest forms of scientific and literary writings to the more modern preoccupation with biological warfare and deadly infirmities such as AIDS, Ebola and the Haanta virus, contagious disease and our collective and individual reactions to it have proven to be a fascinating topic. Although modern science can now successfully identify the pathology and appropriate prophylactic measures to be taken against virtually all known deadly communicable diseases, it is important to recognize that our ability to do so is a relatively modern development. In fact, with regard to the Black Death of 1348–1349, it was not until the late-nineteenth century that scientific epidemiology was able to identify the plague bacillus, Yersinia pestis (formerly known as Pasteurella pestis), as the true culprit behind such widespread mortality.[1] Faced with the task of having to convincingly explain the plague outbreaks of the Iberian peninsula that began in 1348 and recurred in a cyclical fashion up to 1431, Spanish writers of both medical and fictional texts turned to earlier well-known accounts of plague outbreaks in ancient Athens and Constantinople.[2] By following the classical models of authors such as Thucydides, who wrote one of the first known plague accounts documenting the fifth century BC plague at Athens, and Procopius, who likewise detailed the disease's effects in the 527–565 AD outbreak at Constantinople, medieval Iberian writers sought to confer greater authority to their own work.[3] This being the case, in order better to understand the innovations of late-fourteenth to mid-fifteenth century plague writers in the Iberian peninsula, it is useful to first detail some of the characteristics of these earlier plague accounts. As we shall see, plague writing as a genre began with Thucydides and was further developed with the accounts of the second plague pandemic by Procipius, John of Ephesus and the church historian, Evagrius Scholasticus.[4] As such, these authors had a substantial effect on all subsequent forms of plague writing.

Mimêsis and Early Historical Plague Writing

Throughout history, there has been considerable attention paid to the effects of the plague pandemic known as the Black Death that attacked Europe with unbridled ferocity from roughly 1347 to 1352. However, as most scholars of plague realize, the great epidemic of the fourteenth to fifteenth centuries was just one acute incident in a series of plague pandemics that began centuries earlier. In *The Peloponnesian War*, Thucydides documents a pestilence in Athens that appears to have wiped out an even higher proportion than that of medieval London during the time of the Black Death.[5] In his opinion, "nowhere was a pestilence remembered as being so virulent or so destructive of life as it was in Athens" (123).[6] This devastation, which began around the year 427 BC, would eventually carry off one third of the entire population of Athenians. So moving is the account of Thucydides that several later poets and historians adopted it as the literary model for the descriptions of plague in their own works. For example,

> Lucretius (...) bases his own account of the Athenian plague at the end of the sixth book of the De rerum natura (vv. 1138–286) very closely upon that of Thucydides, and Virgil follows suit in this portrayal of a cattle plague in Italy in the third book of the Georgics (478ff). Amongst historians, Diodorus Siculus and Procopius might be singled out especially. The former follows Thucydides not only in his own account of the Athens plague (World History XII, 45 and 58), but also employs him as his model when describing the epidemic which befell the Carthaginians investing Syracuse in 387 BC (ibid XIV, 70.4–72). (Longrigg, 27)

It is also no surprise that Procopius, the historian during the reign of Justinian, adopts Thucydides as his immediate model while documenting the second plague pandemic at Constantinople in AD 542–543. This second pandemic, and the pattern of recurrent epidemics that continue well into the seventh century, is a phenomenon that is described not only by Procopius but also by John of Ephesus and Evagrius Scholasticus.[7] Arguably as destructive as the later plague of the Middle Ages, the so-called "Plague of Justinian" is reported to have caused widespread damage, ultimately reducing the population "40–50 percent by the end of the century" (Russell, 174). The parallels in the writings of those that document this second pandemic—as well with as Thucydides who documents the first—is striking in comparison with what we will later see in the medical and literary plague writing of medieval Spain. Unified in their description of the physical effects, the general disintegration of society and the overall ineffectiveness of the medical practitioner's ability to combat the disease, the writers who document these two earlier pandemics directly mirror the themes we will see repeated in the post-Black Death writings of the Iberian Peninsula.

In one of the only accounts to have survived that contemporaneously documents the first of the three plague pandemics, Thucydides has long been recognized as the model for many subsequent forms of plague writing. In Longrigg's view, such imitation by later authors such as Lucretius and Procopius is "the most sincere form of flattery" as it recognizes the artistic skill of Thucydides in creating such a moving account of the sufferings of the Athenians in their beleaguered city (27). His organization, now accepted as the standard for all plague accounts, begins with the establishment of a specific time frame of the first known incident of plague, a suggestion as to its possible causes—including a suggestion of the poisoning of wells that was a common thought in the years of the Black Death—and the apparent inability of the medical profession to either prevent or cure the infirmity. Thucydides documents that the Peloponnesian War broke out in 431 BC and it is in the summer of the second year of that war that the first known outbreak of plague is reported to have occurred (123). The Peloponnesians, invading Attica and laying waste to the countryside, had forced the peasants to seek refuge within the Long Walls. In Thucydides' estimation, it is this condition of overcrowding that made conditions ripe plague which—after its sudden appearance—spread quickly and killed indiscriminately.

> They [the Peloponnesians and their allies] had not been many days in Attica before the plague first broke out among the Athenians. (…) The plague originated, so they say, in Ethiopia in upper Egypt, and spread from there into Egypt itself and Libya and much of the territory of the King of Persia. In the city of Athens it appeared suddenly, and the first cases were among the population of Piraeus, so that it was supposed by them that the Peloponnesians had poisoned the reservoirs. Later, however, it appeared also in the upper city, and by this time the deaths were greatly increasing in number. (123)

While Thucydides openly admits to lacking the formal medical training to adequately "explain its [the plague's] powerful effects on nature," he does, in fact, spend considerable time in describing the physical effects of the disease (123).

> (…) there seemed to be no reason for the attacks. People in perfect health suddenly began to have burning feelings in the head; their eyes became red and inflamed; inside their mouths there was bleeding from the throat and tongue, and the breath became unnatural and unpleasant. The next symptoms were sneezing and hoarseness of voice, and before long the pain settled on the chest and was accompanied by coughing. Next the stomach was affected with stomach-aches and with vomitings of every kind of bile that has been given a name by the medical profession, all this being accompanied by great pain and difficulty. In most cases there were attacks of ineffectual retching, producing violent spasms; this sometimes ended with this stage of the disease, but sometimes continued long afterwards. Externally the body was not very hot to the touch, nor was their any pallor: the skin was rather reddish and livid, breaking out into small pustules and ulcers. But inside there was a feeling of burning, so that people could not bear the touch even of the lightest linen clothing, but wanted to be completely naked, and indeed most of all would have liked to plunge into cold water. Many of the sick who were uncared for actually did so, plunging into the water-tanks in an effort to relieve a thirst which was unquenchable; for it was just the same with them whether they drank much or little. Then all the time they were afflicted with insomnia and the desperate feeling of not being able to keep still. In the period when the disease was at its height, the body, so far from wasting away, showed surprising powers of resistance to all the agony, so that there was still some strength left on the seventh or

eighth day, which was the time when, in most cases, death came from the internal fever. (124)

Thus describing the general features of the disease, an illness which he reportedly also contracted but ultimately survived, Thucydides then turns the discussion to the social problems directly attributed to the biological disaster.[8]

Throughout his narration, Thucydides makes repeated claims that neither members of the medical profession nor of the clergy are able to either prevent or cure the disease. In fact, he even goes so far as to say that high death rates among the medics and the ineffectiveness of religion actually leads to the avoidance of following either practice.

> At the beginning the doctors were quite incapable of treating the disease because of their ignorance of the right methods. In fact mortality among the doctors was the highest of all. Equally useless were prayers made in the temples, consultation of oracles, and so forth; indeed, in the end people were so overcome by their sufferings that they paid no further attention to such things. (123)

He goes on to describe a state of utter despair in which the fears of deadly contamination far outweighed any sort of individual moral or social obligation.

> Some died in neglect, some in spite of every possible care being taken of them. As for a recognized method of treatment, it would be true to say that no such thing existed: what did good in some cases did harm in others. Those with naturally strong constitutions were no better able than the weak to resist the disease, which carried away all alike, even those who were treated and dieted with the greatest care. The most terrible thing of all was the despair into which people fell when they realized that they had caught the plague; for they would immediately adopt an attitude of utter hopelessness, and, by giving in in this way, would lose their powers of resistance. Terrible, too, was the sight of people dying like sheep through having caught the disease as a result of nursing others. This indeed caused more deaths than anything else. For when people were afraid to visit the sick, then they died with no one to look after them; indeed, there were many houses in which all the inhabitants perished through lack of any attention. When, on the other hand, they did visit the sick, they lost their own lives, and this was particularly true of those who made it a point of honour to act properly. (125–126)

Similar to what we will see in chapters two and three of this investigation that discuss the effects of medieval plague in the Iberian Peninsula and the human reactions to it, not only did this first pandemic result in breakdowns at the individual level where the healthy no longer care for the sick, but it also caused widespread chaos at the greater social level where a state of lawlessness and general debauchery prevailed.

As in the post-Black Death reactions to plague in the Iberian Peninsula, widespread and unpredictable mortality attributed to the Plague of Athens eventually resulted in a breakdown of society which leads to a general state of lawlessness. As we will discuss further in chapter three, such mayhem is directly related to a diminished value of human life due, in part, by the neglecting of funerary ceremonies. A direct result of both the fear of contamination and the abandonment of duties by the clergy due to death or flight, Thucydides draws attention to the fact that the great amounts of deaths due to plague far overwhelm any social mechanisms in place that would perform death ceremonies and, ultimately, dispose of the corpse. As such, the bodies lined the streets and general indiscretions with regard to funerary practices ensued.

> (...) though there were many dead bodies lying about unburied, the birds and animals that eat human flesh either did not come near them or, if they did taste the flesh, died of it afterwards. (...) A factor which made matters much worse than they were already was the removal of people from the country into the city, and this particularly affected the incomers. There were no houses for them, and, living as they did during the hot season in badly ventilated huts, they died like flies. The bodies of the dying were heaped one on top of the other, and half-dead creatures could be seen staggering about in the streets or flocking around the fountains in their desire for water. The temples in which they took up their quarters were full of the dead bodies of people who had died inside them. For the catastrophe was so overwhelming that men, not knowing what would happen next to them, became indifferent to every rule of religion or of law. All the funeral ceremonies which used to be observed were now disorganized, and they buried the dead as best they could. Many people, lacking the necessary means of burial because so many deaths had already occurred in their households, adopted the most shameless methods. They would arrive first at a funeral pyre that had been made by others, put their own dead upon it and set it alight; or, finding another pyre burning, they would throw the

corpse that they were carrying on top of the other one and go away. (125–126)

In Thucydides' view, such disregard of funerary practices combined with the human being's inability to prevent or cure the disease to lead to a general decline in the perceived value of human life. As a result, general lawlessness followed.

L. Fabian Hirst has observed that a common reaction of the collective psychology in the grip of a fatal epidemic is one that results in the extremes of great piety and also great lawlessness.

> From the time of the Attic plague recorded by Thucydides onwards, the great epidemics have evoked a similar response in the herd mind. On the one hand, we see a turning to God with prayers and vows and the dedication of new altars; on the other, a return to ancient, almost forgotten rites and reckless abandonment to riotous living. The belief in demons and evil spirits gains a firmer hold on the popular mind. There is a serious decline in public morale and an increase in crime; especially in robbery and violence inn the cities from which the responsible authorities have fled. Why fear punishment at the hands of man if, tomorrow, one is in any case condemned to die? Pity and sorrow give way to heartless desertion of relatives and friends. (17)

Such is the case of the first plague pandemic where Thucydides describes the unbridled license and drunken merriment that eventually takes the place of piety.

> In other respects also Athens owed to the plague the beginnings of a state of unprecedented lawlessness. Seeing how quick and abrupt were the changes of fortune which came to the rich who suddenly died and to those who had previously been penniless but now inherited their wealth, people now began openly to venture on acts of self-indulgence which before then they used to keep dark. Thus they resolved to spend their money quickly and to spend it on pleasure, since money and life alike seemed equally ephemeral. As for what is called honour, no one showed himself willing to abide by its laws, so doubtful was it whether one would survive to enjoy the name for it. It was generally agreed that what was both honourable and valuable was the pleasure of the moment and everything that might conceivably contribute to that pleasure. No fear of god or law of man had a restraining influence. As for the gods, it seemed to be the same thing whether one worshipped them or not, when one saw the good and the bad dying indiscriminately. As for offences against human law, no one expected to live

> long enough to be brought to trial and punished: instead everyone felt that already a far heavier sentence had been passed on him and was hanging over him, and that before the time for its execution arrived it was only natural to get some pleasure out of life. (126–127)

Thus, faced with the evident truth that religious exercises had failed to protect them against the march of the disease, many people decided that if life was to be short, at least it could be merry. Such a reaction, while frequently noted in the account of Thucydides, was also a common feature in the second pandemic as described by Procopius and Evagrius Scholasticus. Consequently, it would also prove to be a typical comment of authors of the Iberian Peninsula who describe the third pandemic of the fourteenth and fifteenth centuries.

With regard to the second plague pandemic that occurred in Byzantium around the fifteenth year of the reign of Emperor Justinian I (c. 541), the majority of documented information that survives comes from the writings of Procopius, John of Ephesus and Evagrius Scholasticus. This instance of the disease, which would also form a cyclical pattern that continued as a series of epidemics well into the seventh century,[9] paralleled both the first pandemic of 427 BC as well as the third pandemic of 1347 AD in a number of ways. While all these authors when taken together paint a more complete picture of the fearsome illness that struck Constantinople in 543 AD, there are clear differences among these three contemporary accounts. According to Pauline Allen, while all descriptions detail similar effects of plague in the East, the three histories differ in the following manner:

> Procopius' is the most systematic report of the symptoms, the Syriac historian John provides the most graphic and emotional account of the effects of the pestilence in Constantinople and Palestine, and Evagrius, who was attacked by plague as a schoolboy, and later lost a wife, several children, a grandchild, and a good number of town and country servants, gives a personal picture of the suffering caused by the plague's random progress in and around Antioch. (6)

However, despite these differences, all accounts are quite similar to one another as well as to what we have seen in Thucydides' description. With their focus on the physical attributes of the disease, the inability of man to combat it and the resulting social disorder that eventually takes place, the writers of this second plague pandemic also dovetail with what we will see in the Spanish plague writers of the fourteenth and fifteenth centuries.

By and large, the longest and most detailed account of the second pandemic comes to us from the prolific writings of Procopius of Caesarea. As such, a study of his work will comprise the majority of our treatment of the second plague pandemic.

The secretary to Justinian's general, Belisarius, Procopius has enjoyed a reputation as "one of the most notable Greek historians of the Later Roman Empire" (Boak, vii). Although he was, indeed, an eyewitness to what is considered to be a bubonic plague pandemic in Constantinople,[10] Procopius openly cites Thucydides as the *locus classicus* of his own account.[11] Thus, it comes as no surprise that his description also begins with the establishment of the specific time frame and geographic progress of the disease, a reference of man's inability to halt its progress and the apparent randomness in the manner in which it infects its victims.

> During these times [c. 542 AD] there was a pestilence, by which the whole human race came near to being annihilated. (...) But for this calamity it is quite impossible either to express in words or to conceive in thought any explanation, except indeed to refer it to God. For it did not come in a part of the world nor upon certain men, nor did it confine itself to any season of the year, so that from such circumstances it might be possible to find subtle explanations of a cause, but it embraced the entire world, and blighted the lives of all men, though differing from one another in the most marked degree, respecting neither sex nor age. For much as men differ with regard to places in which they live, or in the law of their daily life, or in natural bent, or in active pursuits, or in whatever else man differs from man, in the case of this disease alone the difference availed naught. (...) It started from the Aegyptians who dwell in Pelusium. Then it divided and moved in one direction towards Alexandria and the rest of Aegypt, and in the other direction it came to Palestine on the borders of Aegypt; and from there it spread over the whole world, always moving forward and travelling at times favourable to it. For it seemed to move by fixed arrangement, and to tarry for a specified time in each country, casting its blight slightly upon none, but spreading in either direction right out to the ends of the world, as if fearing lest some corner of the earth might escape it.[12]

Likewise, there is great similarity to Thucydides in the amount of detail and space that Procopius pays to the description of the physical characteristics of the disease. Here, the resemblance of Procopius' description with that of his predecessor is uncanny.

> They [plague victims] had a sudden fever, some when just roused from sleep, others while walking about, and others while otherwise engaged, without any regard to what they were doing. And the body showed no change from the previous colour, nor was it hot as might be expected when attacked by a fever, nor indeed did any inflammation set in, but the fever was of such a languid sort from its commencement and up till evening that neither to the sick themselves nor to a physician who touched them would it afford any suspicion of danger. It was natural, therefore, that not one of those who had contracted the disease expected to die from it. But on the same day in some cases, in others on the following day, and in the rest not many days later, a bubonic swelling developed; and this took place not only in the particular part of the body which is called "boubon" [i.e. groin], that is, below the abdomen, but also inside the armpit, and in some cases also beside the ears, and at different points on the thighs. (...) And when water chanced to be near, they wished to fall into it, not so much because of a desire for drink (for the most rushed into the sea), but the cause was to be found chiefly in the diseased state of their minds. They also had great difficulty in the matter of eating, for they could not easily take food. And many perished through lack of any man to care for them, for they were either overcome by hunger, or threw themselves down from a height. (559–461)

While demonstrating clear similarities to the text of Thucydides in the focus on the random communicability, cold fever and insatiable thirst of the victims, Procopius also comments on what he considers to be another important occurrence in the time of plague. Namely, the apparent inability of humans to prevent or cure the disease through the use of medicine or prayer.

In comparison with the text of Thucydides, the account of Procopius also begins its discussion of the effects of pestilential disease in Byzantium by referring to the impotence of the medical profession in either preventing or curing the infection. Here, his distaste of physical approaches to counter the affliction is almost palpable.

> Now in the case of all other scourges sent from Heaven some explanation of a cause might be given by daring men, such as the many theories

> propounded by those who are clever in these matters; for they love to conjure up causes which are absolutely incomprehensible to man (451)

The equating of the medical practice with an almost profane witch-like notion of "conjuring" serves to illustrate the point that he believes that the plague cannot be understood by means of human reasoning. Later, this idea is reinforced by the inability of physicians to understand even the most basics of the disease's pathology.

> Moreover I am able to declare this, that the most illustrious physicians predicted that many would die, who unexpectedly escaped entirely from suffering shortly afterwards, and that they declared that many would be saved, who were destined to be carried off almost immediately. So it was that in this disease there was no cause which came within the province of human reasoning; for all the cases the issue tended to be something unaccountable. For example, while some were helped by bathing, others were harmed in no less degree. And of those who received no care many died, but others, contrary to reason, were saved. And again, methods of treatment showed different results with different patients. Indeed the whole matter may be stated thus, that no device was discovered by man to save himself, so that either by taking precautions he should not suffer, or that when the malady had assailed him he should get the better of it; but suffering came without warning and recovery was due to no external cause. (463)

Once again recalling the comments of Thucydides, the ineffectiveness of the medical profession is another frequent characteristic that we will see in the post-Black Death writings of the Iberian Peninsula.

Finally, in what is perhaps the most interesting point in the account of Procopius is his report on the social disruption resulting from the disease. Interestingly, while he does correspond with Thucydides—as well as what we will see take place later in the Iberian Peninsula—in the description of various individual reactions that occur because of plague-related fears, Procopius' eyewitness account has a certain supernatural component. As a prelude to the contraction of the disease, Procopius claims that many people "saw supernatural beings either in a waking vision or a dream" (Beatty, 45). It is only when these apparitions would not vanish with the "uttering of the holiest of names," that citizens either fled to the monasteries or isolated themselves in their homes.

> Apparitions of supernatural beings in human guise of every description were seen by many persons, and those who encountered them thought that they were struck by the man they had met in this or that part of the body, as it happened, and immediately upon seeing this apparition they were seized also by the disease. Now at first those who met these creatures tried to turn them aside by uttering the holiest of names and exorcising them in other ways as well as each one could, but they accomplished absolutely nothing, for even in the sanctuaries where the most of them fled for refuge they were dying constantly. But later on they were unwilling even to give heed to their friends when they called to them, and they shut themselves up in their rooms and pretended that they did not hear, although their doors were being beaten down, fearing, obviously, that he who was calling was one of those demons. (455–457)

Despite the novelty of this new supernatural aspect, the account of Procopius continues to echo the social chaos that characteristically accompanies prolonged bouts of plague. Above all, this disorder is most apparent in the treatment of burial rites and social obligations.

> Now in the beginning each man attended to the burial of the dead of his own house, and these they threw even into the tombs of others, either escaping detection or using violence; but afterwards confusion and disorder everywhere became complete. For slaves remained destitute of masters, and men who in former times were very prosperous were deprived of the service of their domestics who were either sick or dead, and many houses became completely destitute of human inhabitants. For this reason it came about that some of the notable men of the city because of the universal destitution remained unburied for many days. (...) And when it came about that all the tombs which had existed previously were filled with the dead, then they dug up all the places about the city one after the other, laid the dead there, each one as he could, and departed; but later on those who were making these trenches, no longer able to keep up with the number of the dying, mounted the towers of the fortifications in Sycae [Modern Galata], and tearing off the roofs threw the bodies in there in complete disorder; and they piled them up just as each one happened to fall, and filled practically all the towers with corpses, and then covered them again with their roofs. As a result of this an evil stench pervaded the city and distressed the inhabitants still more, and especially whenever the wind blew fresh from that quarter. At that time all the customary rites of burial were overlooked. For the dead were not carried out escorted by a procession in the customary manner, nor were the usual chants sung over them, but it was sufficient if one carried on his shoulders the body of one of the dead to the parts of the city which were bordered on the sea and flung him down; and there the

corpses would be thrown upon skiffs in a heap, to be conveyed wherever it might chance. (465–469)

Typical to what we have seen in the account of the first plague pandemic by Thucydides, the overwhelming amount of deaths caused by plague eventually led to an increase in "villainy and in lawlessness of every sort" (471). As we will see in chapters two and three, such an occurrence is also a common reaction noted in the plague writings of medieval Spain.

Past histories of both the first plague pandemic of the fifth century BC and the second plague pandemic of 527–565 AD have, indeed, shaped the perceptions of not only the third pandemic of the fourteenth and fifteenth centuries, but also of modern views with regard to disease as in the case of AIDS. Paul Slack, a scholar who has also studied profiles of different epidemic episodes, also recognizes how intellectual responses to different lethal diseases share a common ancestry in these earlier plague writers. In his view,

> It is notable how Thucydides's description of the plague of Athens (...) produces echoes again and again in literary depictions of later epidemics, some of whose authors may have had access to the Greek historian or to writers who borrowed from him, from Lucretius onwards. Hence, one can never be entirely sure about the extent to which chroniclers of epidemics concentrated on social dislocation, the failure of doctors, flights to and from religion, rumours of poisoned wells, and similar phenomena simply because Thucydides and later writers down to Defoe taught them to look for them. (9)

Having detailed the major characteristics of the accounts of the two earlier plague pandemics, this study can now turn to the consideration of the medical and imaginative writings that took place in the years following the Black Death in medieval Spain. What we will demonstrate is that these later texts will, indeed, show some of the same traits that have been highlighted in the texts of Thucydides and Procopius.

Notes

1. According to Hirst, it is only in the year 1897 that some of the closest scientific observers of plague began to identify the plague bacillus and link the mode of disease transmission with the common black rat. In 1894, new bacteriological techniques allowed for both Professor S. Kitasoto and Dr. A. Yersin to almost simultaneously identify a new kind of bacillus in the blood and tissues of plague patients (106–107). Furthermore, in 1897, independent studies by E.H. Hankin and the French pioneer epidemiologist, P.L. Simond, began to investigate the theory of plague bacilli transmission through breach of the epithelium into the body of man or animal. Simond, the better known proponent of such theories, delivered his findings in a watershed paper in the *Annals of the Pasteur Institute* of Paris in October 1989 (Hirst, 152–153).
2. To clarify our terminology, this study refers to the word 'plague' in accordance with the modern definition--a reference to the specific bacterial strain, *Yersinia pestis*. In contrast, Graham Twigg tells us that "the word plague is derived from the Latin *plaga*, meaning a blow or a stroke, ... but as a word referring to a specific bacterial disease, said to be bubonic plague, it was not used until the seventeenth century. Therefore, the term plague, when used earlier than this in English and Spanish accounts or in translations from Greek or Latin, cannot be accepted as referring specifically to bubonic plague unless there is clear confirmatory evidence" (30). There is also this same liberal use of the term *peste* in Spanish in that it is often used to describe diseases like Spanish influenza, syphilis and even leprosy.
3. Despite substantial controversy with regard to the years surrounding these earlier pandemics, most scholars generally agree in these estimates as taken from Élisabeth Carpentier "The Plague as Recurrent Phenomenon," *The Black Death: a Turning Point in History?* Ed. William M. Bowsky (New York: Holt, Rinehart and Winston, 1971): 35–37.
4. The unavailability of John of Ephesus' text in translation unfortunately makes a direct study impossible. However, useful secondary comments on this text may be obtained in Pauline Allen, "The 'Justinianic' Plague," *Byzantion* 49 (1979), 5–20.
5. See Longrigg, 21. It must be noted that there is some controversy as to whether the first pandemic was actually caused by plague. Lacking specific bacterial evidence to confirm the existence of this specific disease, scholars such as W. P. Macarthur ("The Medical Identification of Some Pestilences of the Past," *Transactions of the Royal Society of Tropical Medicine and Hygiene* 53 (1959), 423–439)

have argued that Thucydides describes an epidemic of typhus fever in Athens. Differing in diagnosis but still denying the existence of plague, R.J. and M.L. Littman conclude the Athenian plague was, in fact, smallpox ("The Athenian Plague: Smallpox," *Transactions of the American Philological Association* 100 (1969), 261–278). However, in one of the most comprehensive studies performed to date, Timothy L. Bratton affirms that "most scholars are agreed that the fearsome illness that struck Constantinople in 543 A.D. was caused by *Yersinia pestis*, the plague bacillus" (part I, 113). He does qualify this statement with the point that it there is still considerable disagreement as to the exact form—bubonic, pneumonic, septicaemic, cutaneous, vesicular or anginal (tonsillar)—of the pestillence.

6. All quotations from Thucydides come from the translation by Rex Warner: Thucydides, *The Peloponnesian War*, Book Two, (Middlesex: Penguin Books, 1954). I cite by page number.

7. See Procopius, *History of the Wars*, Books I and II, Trans. H.B. Dewing (London: William Heinemann, 1914): 450–473; John of Ephesus, *Joannis Episcopi Ephesi Syri Monophysitae Commentarii de Beatis Orientalibus et Historiae Ecclesiasticae Fragmenta*, Trans. W.J. Van Douwen and J.P.N. Land (Amsterdam: Verhandelingen der Koninklijke Akademie van Nederland, 1889): 227–40; Evagrius Scholasticus, "Ecclesiastical History of Evagrius," *History of the Church by* Theodoret *and* Evagrius, (London: Henry G. Bohn, 1854): 408–413.

8. The idea that Thucydides himself was stricken by plague is based on his own statement which serves as a preface to his listing of the disease's features: "I caught the disease myself and observed others suffering from it" (22). For this statement to be true, it is generally assumed that the author was in Athens in 430 BC. However, one should not overlook Longrigg's theory that "he might have contracted the disease in the north when it was brought to Thrace by Hagnon's troops sent to reinforce those beseiging Potidaea. It may be recalled that Thucydides had an estate and gold-mining concessions in Thrace and much of his military service seems to have been located there" (27). No matter the case, it is clear that Thucydides must have had first-hand knowledge of the disease as his account is so specific in terms of details.

9. For a detailed summary of the periodicity of the epidemic waves of the second plague pandemic, see J.N. Biraben and Jacques Le Goff, "The Plague in the Early Middle Ages," *Biology of Man in History*, Ed. Robert Forster and Orest Ranum (Baltimore: Johns Hopkins UP, 1975): 48–80.

10. That this major plague was strictly bubonic is still a point of debate among some scholars. For a comprehensive review of scholarly opinion on the subject, see Timothy L. Bratton, "The Identity of the Plague of Justinian," *Transactions and Studies of the College of Physicians of Philadelphia*, vol. 3.2 (June 1981), 113, n. 1.

11. It must be noted that imitation—or *mimêsis*—was common practice in Byzantine literature. Thus, the idea of Procopius using Thucydides as a historical model would not have seemed out of place for "such imitation was effectively dictated by the educational system of the Roman empire, where stress was laid exclusively on a backward-looking study and reworking of a fixed canon of the classics, with low value being attached to originality" (Cameron, 33). Indeed, the serious historian who wished to give an authoritative tone to his work could not avoid such imitation. Procopius, then, would have necessarily followed his model in the use of language—specifically vocabulary and sentence structure—as well as in the organization and presentation of content.

12. All quotations from Procopius follow the pagination as found in: Procopius, *History of the Wars* II, Trans. H.B. Dewing (London: William Heinemann, 1914), with page numbers in parenthesis.

• CHAPTER TWO •
Medical Writing / Treatises of Medieval Spain

> This is an example of the wonderful deeds and power of God, because never before has a catastrophe of such extent and duration occurred. No satisfactory reports have been given about it, because the disease is new (...) God only knows when it will leave the earth. (Medical Writer Ibn Khatimah, Andalusia: 1349)[1]

In comparison with the writers such as Thycydides and Procopius who documented the first pandemic of the fifth century BC and the second pandemic of the sixth century AD, the Spanish writers of the third pandemic that reaches the Iberian Peninsula in 1348 treat the discussion of the disease in a new manner. Due in part to advancements in scientific thought along with significant changes in the perceptions that Spanish physicians had about their role in society, fourteenth-century medical writers broke the tradition of earlier writers such as Thucydides and Procopius—who constructed their work around the physical description of plague—and began to write in more preventative manners.[2] Medical texts, noting the cyclical nature of plague that re-occurred throughout an individual's lifetime, began to address the disease in terms of proactive measures—such as a modified diet or change in daily habits—that, if followed, would successfully stave off the disease. In this respect, such Spanish authors felt the need to do more than just serve as writers of historical documentaries that recorded the chaos only after the outbreak. This fundamental change in the role of medical texts did not occur arbitrarily at this moment in time. Rather, a gradual change can be seen as a direct result of the shifting perceptions in science, a consequence of the scourge of pestilential disease in medieval Spain.

Guy Beaujouan, commenting on the numerous factors that affected the development of science in the Iberian Peninsula, concluded that the late Middle Ages was characterized by a general weakness of scientific study at the Spanish universities.[3] Physicians of the fourteenth century who wished to study at the leading schools at the time were forced to seek their education at one of the six principal medical schools in Europe: Salerno, Montpellier, Bologna, Paris, Padua and Oxford.[4] Because of close contact with nearby Arabic, Byzantine and, later, Jewish physicians, the faculty members at these medical schools began to stress the innovative concept of understanding human infirmities through a greater study of anatomy. Despite the fact that the initial corporal-based studies were founded on the dissection and understanding of pig physiology, this change was, nonetheless, a milestone in the evolution of scientific thought. Combined with the fact that a disproportionate number of the practicing physicians and surgeons—as a consequence of being in close contact with the afflicted—were themselves ultimately victims of the plague, the time period surrounding the Black Death was ripe for bringing about widespread changes in medical theory and practice.[5] Above all, these changes can be seen in the medical texts themselves as they were a primary vehicle in the dissemination of medical information.

Jon Arrizabalaga recognized in his study of the Black Death in the Crown of Aragon that university medical practitioners were not the only citizens who sought to treat medical conditions such as plague:

> In fact, this battle was waged by *all* the people concerned with health activities: both by those educated in the universities, and by those trained in the 'open' system: ordinary men and women, Jews, Muslims and Christians—and by many who would be classified today as 'quacks.' (238)

With the ever-increasing number of university trained medical practitioners becoming, themselves, victims of plague, those that we would now consider "outside" medical practitioners—such as local barbers, midwives and medically inclined everyday citizens—took up the slack in addressing their society's medical needs.[6] As such, the university trained medical practitioner began to write to this new audience. As a result, the medical practitioners changed their focus from simple descriptions of plague, those that focused on documenting symptoms, to an approach in which instruction in precautionary measures and cures were of central importance so as to be of use to the "outside" medical practitioner. With this new intended audience in mind, medical texts began to be written in a clearer manner that could be easily understood by the common man. They also needed to prescribe specific procedures to healers that were typically not educated in the university. In addition, they needed to communicate their counsel to the governing bourgeoisie and to the political authorities governing the municipalities. This new interest in a clinical approach to plague reflects an ideological change in Spain that was unknown until the late thirteenth and fourteenth century.

Before one can comprehend the innovations in this first stage of clinically oriented plague writing that emerges during and following the Black Death in the Iberian Peninsula, it is useful to detail some of the older theories of pre-plague medicine. As we shall see, one of the most important legacies of plague in Europe as a whole was the destruction of existing medical systems that based its practice on the ideas of Hippocrates, Galen and Arabic theorists such as the Persian Avicenna.[7]

Prior to 1347, the structural division of professionals in the medical field reflected the medieval concept of trifunctionalism.

> At the top were physicians. They were elite, highly trained in current theories of medicine, small in number and very exclusive; they were accorded a degree of respect and prestige in keeping with their role as the paramount authorities. They were the heirs to Hippocrates and Galen. Physicians were always men and, in northern Europe, usually members of the clergy. This religious connection was important, part of an association of medicine and religion extending to the Biblical world and, no doubt, beyond, in which the power to heal was associated with first magic, then the supernatural, and finally, special religious gifts. As a result, medieval medical education was generally connected with and supervised by the church. (Gottfried, 105).

As a direct result of having been professionally trained in an academic medical environment, it was the medical physician—as opposed to the surgeon or other lesser medical practitioners—who was publicly acknowledged as more valuable to his profession and to ordinary life.[8] This being the case, when the Black Death initially entered the peninsula and began its swift progression towards the Mediterranean coast, it befell the university educated medical physician to give the necessary scientific instruction that outside medical practitioners could employ in their attempt to prevent and cure pestilential infection. Lacking sufficient qualified medical physicians for establishing mentoring programs through which to personally disseminate necessary medical information, the medical text, and its ability to give practical advice concerning plague, assumed a paramount importance. According to Arrizabalaga,

> (…) their interpretations of the nature and causes of the Black Death, a well as the measures they suggested to keep their fellow citizens healthy and the (very few) remedies to cure those who were taken ill with pestilence, represent the earliest responses made by professionals trained at the rising university medical faculties to a scourge which would not leave Western Europe until the eighteenth century, as well as the first steps towards the construction of this disaster as a disease-entity. (286)

Before the Black Death, this sort of practical advice was nonexistent. Originally directed to other medical practitioners and wealthy individuals such as royalty, or civil and ecclesiastical nobility, new purposes in writing would evolve to form a medical literary genre of its own called in Latin *regimen sanitatis*: health and its preservation.[9]

Prior to the Black Death, medical theory and the understanding of health throughout Europe was based on the theory of the humors. Essentially, this theory held that the body had four basic humors: blood, phlegm, yellow bile, and black bile which, in turn, all had unique characteristics and corresponded to particular internal organs:

> Blood came from the heart, phlegm from the brain, yellow bile from the liver, and black bile from the spleen. Galen and Avicenna attributed certain elemental qualities to each humor. Blood was hot and moist, like air; phlegm was cold and moist, like water; yellow bile was hot and dry, like fire; and black bile was cold and dry, like earth. In effect, the human body was a microcosm of the larger world. (Gottfried, 106)

When one could successfully maintain balance among the four basic humors, this state was known as *Eukrasia*. Conversely, human sickness reflected a condition known as *Dyskrasia*, where the body's humors were not in equilibrium. It was, in turn, the task of the medical practitioner to diagnose the imbalance causing illness in an individual and prescribe the appropriate remedy—or remedies—for restoring the balance of the humors to the patient.

Compared to modern standards of medical treatment, the manner in which the fourteenth century medical practitioner attempted to correct the condition of *Dyskrasia* might seem primitive. However, by the time of the Black Death in Europe, healing of the sick still followed the lines proposed by ancient Greek and Islamic theorists.

> The diffusion of the *Isagoge* of Iohannitius—one of the writings contained in the *Articella*—throughout the twelfth and thirteenth centuries introduced into European learned circles its famous threefold organization of medicine's subject matter into naturals (things forming a part of living beings, such as elements, humours, qualities, and complexions), the contranaturals (things inimical to life and health, such as disease, causes of disease, and symptoms), and the nonnaturals (a set of things necessary for life and affecting the condition of the body). The nonnaturals were organized under six headings: (1) air (and environment), (2) motion and rest, (3) food and drink, (4) sleep and waking, (5) evacuation and repletion (including sexuality), and (6) affections of the soul. (García-Ballester, 121)

In *Techne iatrike*, Galen affirmed that it was through proper management of the regimen of the patient that health or the avoidance of disease could be effected. Consequently, texts on the art of medicine were chiefly concerned with altering the non-natural factors as "a way to balance the four basic qualities (hot, cold, moist and dry) and thus to affect the character of the humours and the state of humoral balance" (Rather, *Six Things*, 339).

Disease, then, was assumed to be directly correlated with some intemperance of man or his immediate environment and it was only through restored temperance that one's physical ailments could be relieved. Of course, the ability to maintain a regulated system of diet or other physical modality was not economically feasible for the majority of the population prior to the Black Death. Control over such external factors was feasible only for those individuals who had the economic or political independence to exercise their freedom of choice and effectively modify their diet or lifestyle. Medical physicians before the Black Death recognized this and, as a result, the implied reader in the majority of their texts was a member of the economic elite. However, pestilential disease and its recurring nature slowly changed the society in which it occurred and, subsequently, enlarged the readership of medical texts as well. The result was a new writing that was more aware of, and took into account, an expanded base of readers and consultants.

In the late thirteenth and well into the fourteenth century, one can clearly identify an ideological change throughout Europe in the concept of medicine and health, a change that comes about from disruptions caused by plague. In 1956, Amada López de Meneses published her *Documentos acerca de la peste negra en los dominios de la corona de Aragón* which vividly detail the economic and political confusion that enveloped King Pedro IV's reign at the time of the Black Death. As reflected in this series of official documents that date from April 20, 1348 to May 4, 1384, the disruption and disorder caused by the plague that ultimately claimed the life of both Pedro IV's wife, Leonor, and youngest daughter, María, had consequences that affected nearly every level of society (López de Meneses, Nos. 11, 38–40). Politically, the administrative sector of the Crown of Aragon was one of the hardest hit and replacing public officials became one of the king's primary concerns. For example, in a document dated July(?) 16(?), 1348, Pedro IV empowered the governor of Rousillon to fill vacancies as best he could since "a consecuencia de la peste fallecieron casi todos los oficiales y notarios de Rosellón y Cerdaña" (López de Menesis, No. 13).[10] Likewise, similar problems quickly broke out in other parts of Aragon. As Melanie Shirk recognizes, the high plague mortality of political officers forced the need to replace them with immediate and often less qualifies substitutes:

> By July (...) Barcelona had lost not only four out of its five city councillors [sic] (No. 28), but almost everyone on the governing Council of One Hundred (Capmany y de Montpalau 1962: 987) (...) At times one official simply exercised several functions, like the attorney for Bas and Castellfollit who was given the further duties of assessor and professor of jurisprudence (López de Meneses 1956: No.51). When all legal officials in Bergá perished, the town's surviving notary had to assume all their jobs (No. 24). The bailiff of Arbucies had to exercise the same function because judges and scribes in nearby Villafranca de Panadés were taking advantage of the scarcity of legal talent to ask 'immoderate fees and expenses' (No. 76). The shortage of professors of jurisprudence proved so serious that, in 1351, the king took the unusual step of extending the terms of office of three attornies [sic] of Perpignan for three years (No. 119). (360)[11]

As royal notaries and other legal officials were commonly in charge of taking down the last testaments of those dying from plague, the dangerously close contact with those infected resulted in an understandably high death toll for members of these groups. In Almudévar, for example, Pedro IV was even forced to legalize documents produced by private citizen Juan de Atraro when "durante la peste negra, fallecidos los notarios, se hizo cargo de la última voluntad testamentaria de los enfermos" (No. 27). Such disorder in the political and legal sectors of society eventually took its toll on the economic stability of the peninsula. The result was a society that experienced the short-term effects of a rapid re-distribution of wealth whereby the rich suffered losses as many of the poor made significant fiscal gains as a consequence of the long-term effects of a general economic restructuring.

As demonstrated in the López de Meneses documents, an almost immediate strain was put on the economic model of the time when the established feudal system degenerated into semi-chaos owing to the effects of the plague. Typical of the majority of Europe immediately preceding the Black Death, Spain had been functioning under a feudal mode of production where the peasant worked a small farm and paid tributes in the form of rents to the lords who owned that land. With the onset of the plague pandemic and the physicians' apparent inability to prevent or cure the disease, large numbers of people who worked the land either fled or succumbed to plague.[12] This immediately produced a decline in agricultural production as farms were left unattended as well as a consequential loss of revenue to the land-owning classes.

> Requests to lower taxes and tributes followed quickly in the wake of the plague, and the king handled them as discretely as the administrative problems. The royal treasury suffered early economic repercussions from the Black Death, and not only was the king unable to grant direct financial aid to his subjects, but his own income was abruptly diminished (...) Taxes and tributes in a number of places had to be waived for up to five years (Nos. 46, 82, 107, 108, 109, 111, 114, 118, 128), while elsewhere fines were reduced or exemptions or remissions were made (Nos. 34, 69, 93). (Shirk, 362)

As a response to the legal confusions that accompanied the high mortality rates of notaries and other administrative professionals, private citizens besieged an already understaffed governmental body with claims and disputes over inheritances. The lack of wills often made it difficult for rightful heirs to obtain their legacies and, often, looters stripped estates of their valuables without fear of justice. On June 7, 1348, a member of the royal house complains of being robbed of "el dinero y los muebles y efectos de su domicilio" in Barcelona after the death of his wife and in-laws (No. 10). Likewise, on February 24, 1349, Pedro IV orders an "investigación del robo" and subsequent "castigo ejemplar" of the culprits who sacked the estate of a landowner who died of plague in Terrassola (No. 57). Finally, a document dated April 7, 1350 orders justice in the case of Pedro Garcés de Vizcarra who,

> durante la peste perdió a su padre y a su hermana, de cuyos bienes se apoderaron gentes del lugar que, alegando parentesco con los difuntos, se negaban a devolver su presa. (No. 99)

Legal disruptions such as these also made it difficult for many lenders to recover losses from the descendants of debtors.[13] In a document dated January 5, 1349, Pedro IV settles such a dispute when he orders that a family that occupies a vacant house in Teruel claiming to be relatives of the deceased "pag[ue] las deudas y cargas correspondientes" that Jewish moneylenders demand of them in default of a loan made to the previous owner (No. 52). It is clear that this was not an isolated case; many similar examples confirm that the political and economic disruptions caused by the plague had similar short-term consequences that either benefited or damaged the livelihood of select individuals. However, in order to understand how plague caused a change in the focus and reception of medical texts, one must look to the disease's long-term consequences.

It has been affirmed by many scholars who study plague in the Middle Ages that had it not been for the Black Death and the pernicious viral outbreaks that would follow, Europe would have never had the impetus to free itself from the feudal system. David Herlihy, one of the most prominent advocates of this viewpoint, summarizes his ideas as follows:

> Europe at about 1300 was a land caught in a Malthusian deadlock, in a demographic and economic situation which paralyzed its capacity to improve the ways it produced its goods. That system, marked by the saturated use of resources and stagnant outputs, might have persisted indefinitely. The plague broke the deadlock, and allowed Europeans to rebuild their demographic and economic systems in ways more admissive of further development. Culturally, the plague thinned the cadres of the

skilled and learned and reduced their years of service; it weakened schools and universities; and it compromised the quality of cultural traditions. (81)[14]

In short, with the Black Death and subsequent plague epidemics keeping the population in check, the dramatic decrease in the number of workers had the long-term effect of driving up the price of wage labor. Seigneurial reserve, a system that was already on the decline by 1347, disappeared in its entirety in many regions. The abandonment of farmland immediately sent prices soaring and while peasants could still provide for the subsistence of their own family in the cultivation of private parcels, the landlords suffered greatly.[15]

> The lords, both lay and ecclesiastical, suffered an unbelievable diminution in revenue from ground rents. Rents dropped by half, sometimes by three-quarters, because of the immense amount of land that was abandoned and because conditions had become very favorable for tenants on the lands that remained in cultivation. Offerings to churches decreased in the same proportion. (Renouard, 30)

For landed proprietors such as nobility and clergy, the situation was often catastrophic especially for the smaller landowner who did not own enough acres of land to weather such dynamic economic conditions.

> Many lords were forced to abandon any form of direct cultivation and lease their entire estates, collecting cash *rentiers* and usually becoming absentee landlords. In an era of rising prices, this could be disastrous, especially when the tenants held the land with long-term copyhold leases. (Gottfried, 138)

As the number of laborers decreased, the bargaining power of those remaining increased to the point of seeing the rise of overly ambitious peasants who enjoyed a standard of living superior to many newly-impoverished gentlemen. This, of course, brought on political and moral attacks condemning the greed and pride of the self-determined peasant. The new situation represented an inversion of the natural order.

> For contemporary chroniclers, the behavior of the lower classes after the plague was a clear sign of the world plunging further into sin. Modern readers, who generally do not share the medieval commitment to social hierarchy as an expression of divine order, are unlikely to agree. In any analysis of the plague's impact the increased bargaining power of workers, and the adjustment of the balance of power between lords and their tenants,

> are now more likely to be seen as benefits. Although these changes were contained with some success in the short term, the recurrence of plague in the 1360s and 1370s made them irresistible. (Horrox, 243)[16]

The cyclical nature of plague resulted in fundamental long-term changes in the lifestyle of the peasant and their bargaining power with their lords. The result was an upper class that could no longer afford some of the luxuries in life and a lower class that now had greater control over their work and their leisure.

The changes in tenurial and agricultural systems had numerous long-term effects but it was the social changes and the decline of traditional systems that was to influence the role of medicine and, subsequently, the function of the medical text. While a fair number of the landowners could clearly no longer afford the luxuries they once had enjoyed—such as personalized medical attention—the serf exercised greater control over his time and labor. For the first time in centuries, low rent prices and underemployment meant that peasants who were unhappy with their work situation could pick up and move to more agreeable circumstances.

> A peasant could leave in the middle of the night, go to the next manor, and expect to be welcomed, so short was the supply of labor. Any lord who hoped to keep his workers had to offer them better terms of tenure than they had had before the Black Death. (Gottfried, 137)

Just as the rural supply of labor had dwindled, recurrent plague outbreaks combined with the denser urban population to cause an even greater shortage of industrial labor in the cities: "se estima que la pestilencia se propagaba con mayor facilidad en los núcleos urbanos, en los que el contagio era mayor que en los rurales" (Valdeón, 22). Although specific demographic data on the years prior to the Black Death are virtually non-existent for the majority of the Iberian Peninsula, workers in the Crown of Aragon took advantage of the demand for labor as seen in the sharp rise in wages circa 1340 in Valencia, Aragon and Navarre. Through extrapolation of the numerous laws enacted within a short time after the Black Death, one finds that wage increases of four and five times their pre-plague level was a problem universal to the entire Iberian Peninsula.[17]

> The same situation existed throughout western Europe and everywhere the monarchies reacted in the same way. To restrain the rise of wages and prices

they sought to prevent free movement of labour. The laws promulgated by the Aragonese Cortes of Saragossa in 1350, those of the Castilian Cortes of 1351, and Portuguese laws of 1349–50 all sought to attain the same object, 'to regulate prices and wages in a sense favourable to employers and consumers, that is essentially the privileged classes, bourgeois of the towns, nobles and ecclesiastics'[18] (Hillgarth, 5)

The effectiveness of laws that attempted to regulate wages and commodity prices was certainly questionable—especially when considering that the legal and juridical sectors of most regions were already suffering from severe shortages of manpower and, thus, were unable to successfully impose such edicts. However, the fact that governments tried at all to address the problem of salaries demonstrates the new advantage that workers possessed due to widespread labor shortages. Subsequent deadly outbreaks eventually forced the revocation of most wage regulating legislation and, by 1352, labor shortages had ultimately conceded superior bargaining power to working-class survivors.

The long-term benefit for the majority of the working-class survivors of the many lethal infections to occur in Medieval Spain was an increase in disposable income, better working conditions and more leisure time. All of these factors eventually produced new interest in and, consequently, new perceptions of health, medicine and the role of the medical caregivers in society. The widespread renegotiation of labor services, while benefiting a good number of workers who continued with their same pre-plague occupation, also allowed many to better their economic standings by changing professions, as regional necessities dictated. While it is clear that many of the poorest in society remain destitute due to the sharp increase in the price of goods at this time, reductions or complete suspensions of rents and taxes provided the economic flexibility for many peasants to dabble in usury as both worker and landowner alike regularly found themselves lacking funds in this unstable economic environment. Due to the decrease in people to work the land efficiently, specialization of crops occurs in many regions while many other land-owners were forced to switch from agricultural production to the less labor-intensive raising of livestock.

In Castile, for example, economic change due to a plague-affected population level brought about the widespread beginning of an industry that exists until today: "la progresión de la ganadería lanar castellana (la oveja merina *hija de la pestilencia*, diría en el siglo XVIII Sarmiento..." (Mitre, 18). Spain, just as the rest of post-plague European community, was slowly becoming more specialized in terms of occupations, agricultural and industrial production. With this change came a greater sense of professional accountability, especially in what the working public demanded of its intellectual elite in the political and medical sectors.

New urban groups such as merchants, craftsmen and professionals in the late medieval Mediterranean cities felt great concern for the economic and social chaos resulting from endemic pestilential disease and demanded immediate relief from city officials. Once only a private concern, the perceptions of health and medicine grew in importance as a social concern. Healthcare was now considered a public good or *publica utilitas*,

> (...) with implications for medicine but also with political repercussions and practical consequences for the everyday life of people. Municipalities, especially the strong in the Crown of Aragon, took the lead in a new sanitary policy, dealing with, among other things, the control of foods (especially meat and fish), the cleaning of streets, the removal of garbage, disputes over pollution of the air (from irritating smoke) or of drinking-water (from liquids oozing out of olive-oil mills), the cultivation of rice fields in marshes, and the control of sanitary officers. (García-Ballester, 120)

Public officials, reacting to the demands of its citizenry for better medical policies dealing with the prevention and cure of recurrent pestilential disease, demanded recommendations from their health-care elite: the medical practitioner. However, as fourteenth century medical practitioners still drew almost all their epidemiological knowledge from the thousand year old *Book of Fevers* by Galen, their joined opinion yielded few practical results and, with their almost exclusive training in medical theory as opposed to experience with human physiology, this is hardly surprising. At the time, the source of the authority by which the medical practitioner exercised his craft was founded largely on psychological bases:

> Everyone felt better when self-confident, expensive experts could be called in to handle a vital emergency. Doctors relieved others of the responsibility for deciding what to do. As such their role was strictly comparable to that of

the priesthood, whose ministrations to the soul relieved anxieties parallel to those relieved by medical ministrations to the body. (McNeill, 209)

Of course, since the medical profession being so closely interrelated with a tangible and empirically measurable reality, the results of their professional advice was more easily assessed; however, more often than not, their professional opinion made little difference. Despite the lack of training in practical anatomy and pathology of the surgeon—considered to be inferior to the practitioner due to their lack of theoretical background—medical practitioners continued to be the primary source of *official* medical opinion.[19] As such, they produced nearly every tractate of medical opinion dealing with medieval plague visitation that exists today. At times similar to and different from one another and from their predecessors in medical literature, these works remain important for two main reasons: 1) they provide insight to the development of medical practice since they document a transition era when medicine began to shift from the private to the public sphere, and 2) they were written under stress during a period of great fear and, as such, offer a glimpse of how man tried to come to terms with such a pernicious calamity.

The selected medical texts that are discussed in the following section are among many that were produced in and around the time of pestilential outbreaks in the Iberian Peninsula. These tractates were chosen because the ideas contained therein are representative of the changing perceptions of the function of medicine and healing initially provoked by the Black Death. Innovative in comparison with ancient texts (Thucydides and Procopius), this new style of medical text focused on preventative measures and cures that could be employed to attempt to contain widespread contagious infection. Common to many medieval works, these medical texts often lack a specific date of composition and, as such, their dating is often contested by specialists. With this in mind, every effort has been made to present these works in chronological order. Although biographical data on their authors is also scarce, such information is included whenever possible.

"Del regimiento en tienpo de pestilencia," *Menor daño de medicina*. Segunda parte del regimiento de sanidat, Capítulo XIII. Alonso de Chirino

The "Regimento en tienpo de pestilencia," by Alonso de Chirino, is the second sub-section of the first volume of a larger collection of manuscripts that goes by the collective title: *Menor daño de medicina*. Although relatively little solid biographical data exists for Chirino, it is generally agreed that his life transpired in Castile between the reigns of Enrique III (reigned 1390–1406) and Juan II (reigned 1406–1454).[20] The exact date of his birth and death is unknown; however María Teresa Herrera finds that it was fairly certain that Chirino lived to know Juan II's eldest son, Enrique IV, until the prince reached age four:

> Enrique IV nace en 1425 y en 1429 Chirino otorga su testamento, muriendo poco después (...) En 1431 un documento existente en el Archivo Histórico de Simancas da cuenta de que Doña Violante López otorga un juro a favor de uno de sus hijos. Si en esta fecha ya había muerto su esposo y la fecha del testamento es la de 1429 puede asegurarse que la muerte debió sobrevenirle entre ambas fechas. (Intro, XV)[21]

Chirino studied and eventually practiced medicine for a short time in Castile when, unexpectedly, he decided to abandon the profession. After suffering negative experiences due to the greediness of his colleagues in medicine who were more concerned with personal wealth than with curing the sick, Chirino abandoned the practice of medicine to travel throughout Castile and Aragon preaching the moral responsibilities of the healing profession. He himself acknowledges this important part of his life:

> Todo esto pregoné e demostré muchas vezes delante de los grandes señores estando ende muchos famosos letrados en los logares mucho públicos, en Castilla e en Aragón en los años de la Natividad de Nuestro Salvador Ihesus Crixto de mil e quatroçientos honze e de doze e treze años fasta que fuí candado de dar bozes tres años. E non fallé boz ni escuchador nin quien lo quisiere bien entender... (Intro, XVI)

It is this disdain of greedy medical practitioners that eventually led to his numerous, albeit ill-received, petitions to Enrique III for regulation and reform of the profession. Eventually, this same personal dedication to the reform of his profession brought him the acclaim of Juan II who named Chirino to his court with the esteemed title: "Alcalde e examinador mayor de los físicos e çirugianos de sus reignos e señoríos" (Intro, XVI).

It is clear that Chirino's personal dedication to speak against deceit and ignorance among those in the medical profession also served as the inspiration for his *Menor daño de medicina*. Although the exact date of composition is unknown, scholars such as María Teresa Herrera believe that this work was written during the later part of the author's life as only one secure in his position could exhibit such unfettered criticism of his colleagues. The title to the second subdivision of his work, "Capítulo primero que muestra que poco saben los físicos en los particulares," illustrates the tone of the entire work (57). In the introduction to this section, Chirino explicitly blames the ignorance of medical practitioners on their lack of clinical study:

> Non es de tachar el dezir o repetir muchas vezes la cosa que ninguna vez non es tomada. Por ende avn quiero repetir que todas las obras de los médicos son dudosas e que curan con / aquellas reglas genrales que fallan en la mediçina e que en los singulares poco es lo que entienden por conosçimiento singular ... E ende caben tantos yerros e dudas que no son numerables, tanto, que mucho por marauilla conteçe ser ninguna çeçión conoçida çierta e acauadamente por ningunt médico nin físico saluo en el dezir. Que muchas palabras se pueden en ello dezir que parescan razones e sienpre con aventura de mentir; por lo qual en esto está más público que vsan en estas / curas de las dichas reglas generales. (57–58)

With the simple desire to try to help patients protect themselves from the dangers of improper medical advice, Chirino set down in writing specific information that he believed could be applied to the population in general. Above all else, his explicit rule is that each individual should employ the remedies he suggests only with regard to their specific situation. He dedicates sections to both the rich as well as the poor detailing how each should modify their daily regimen to best accommodate the excess or lack of medicinal resources inherent to their social class. He advocates the use of natural cures over medicine whenever possible and also warns of using medicine that is old or unproven by clinical experimentation. Finally, and most importantly, he warns against blindly following the advice of medical authorities:

> Por ende non vos aquexedes faziendo muchas melezinas o pensando quel físico sabe más que vos que poco es aquello que sabe. (8)

Although he indeed recognizes the value of having a qualified professional personally evaluate a given medical condition, Chirino is also quick to denounce the many physicians who merely give an authoritative tone to useless and outdated, albeit popular, medical treatments.

Conforming to the general expectations of most post-Black Death medical tractates in terms of organization of pertinent topics, the *Menor daño de medicina* is divided into the following larger sections or "partes:" the first grouping deals with the health regiment and how the reader can stave off sickness with proper food, drink and exercise; the second section treats the cures for general health issues; and the third discusses appropriate remedies and surgeries to correct specific disorders. Of these three areas, it is clear that the author follows the new post-Black Death trend in giving greater weight to the role of a strict health regiment in the prevention of illness. In a prologue to the entire work, Chirino openly acknowledges this importance:

> Pero que la más loada parte es la del regimiento de sanidat porque non ay en ello peligro ninguno e puede auer grant prouecho. E el curar de las enfermedades puede auer peligro en lo quel físico faze tan bien commo sanar. (12)

Keeping with the idea of providing a health regimen that is as safe as possible, Chirino affirms that the data provided in his work are "las más seguras que non trayan peligro" and that the advice given is the same that he would give to a friend (12).

Obviously, as an author Chirino is aware that the reader of his material is also the prospective patient. Such a form of medical writing in which the intended recipient was not someone trained in basic health procedures was virtually non-existent in Spain before 1347. Chirino is conscious of this fact and, as a result, he constructs his work by reducing every medical concept to the simplest of terms. He initially addresses this goal in the prologue with a statement he directs towards the reader:

> (...) todo lo que aqui fallardes escripto non será por vocablos de medeçina nin por palabras escuras saluo fablando bulgarmente que qualquier omne puede entender. (6)

Although he does, in fact, avoid the use of medical terminology, whenever such vocabulary is unavoidable Chirino takes extra steps to explain troublesome words in the simplest terms possible. For example, to differentiate between the different forms of "çiçiones" so as to advise on the proper treatment, Chirino is careful to describe specific symptoms and reactions of those afflicted with each individual strain of the illness. The "çiçión de flema" then is explained as that "que viene cada día con frío a los pies et a las otras estremidades o con espeluzamiento / e frío en las espaldas e a menester cobrirse de rropa" (60). Such explanations—whereby the author gives two or three synonymous descriptions of the same concept—could hardly have been misunderstood by the reader and once the idea was understood, the proper treatment was sure to be administered.

In what specifically concerns the treatment of plague, Chirino is particularly vocal. If one accepts the dating of the author's biography, it is clear that plague still had a grip on the Iberian Peninsula both during the author's life as well as when his work was circulated. This being the case, it is not surprising that the topic of pestilence takes up an overwhelming majority of the entire tractate. As its inclusion in the first part of the *Menor daño de la medicina* would indicate, the larger part of this section deals with the proper health regimen to follow for success in the prevention of the disease. However, as Carreras Panchón points out in his study of the loimological texts of the Spanish Renaissance,

> (...) los conceptos de prevención y tratamiento del mal se confunden siendo difícil establecer una separación neta entre los remedios que se consideran preservativos y los curadores. (91)

Similar to the popular Spanish proverb, "Huir de la pestilencia con tres eles es prudencia: luego, lexos y luengo tiempo," the fundamental recommended act of prevention was physical distance: "Lo prinçipal es salir de aquella tierra onde se cabsa o está cabsada la pestilençia e lo más ante que pudiere" (39). Curiously, the recommendations to those faced with the inability to escape direct contact with the inflicted is nearly the same as the advice Chirino gives to those who have already contracted the disease. To both groups, the author suggests moderation in the intake of heavy foods such as meat and dairy products while increasing the intake of bitter foodstuffs:

> El vinagre e todas cosas agras e toda vianda onde se pueda poner miel e vinagre, que sea más agro que dulçe, e çerrajas e borrajas e todas frutas agras e ásperas e agraz e su arrope. E granadas e mançanas agras e las lentejas con miel e vinagre o en qualquier manera, son buenas para esto. (39–40)

In conformity with the precepts of humoral theory, it is also recommended that one be mindful of bad "ayres" and that when noxious odors are detected, "conuiene cada día safumar la moradea e çerca de sí mesmo con ençienso" (41). However, despite its intent to offer worthwhile medical advice on both the prevention as well as cure of plague, it is clear by the greater focus on preventative measures that Chirino is more optimistic about this part of his medical advice. Perhaps indicative of his own grim prognosis for those who actually contract the disease, the last chapter in this section ends on a spiritual rather than physical note.

While Chirino's treatise on the prevention and cure of pestilential disease does, ultimately, contain a great deal of solid medical advice based on the new post-Black Death concepts of health and medicine, one must recognize that science had experienced severe shortcomings during that period. Despite the efforts of the many who practiced medicine, plague still remained an uncontrollable virus that usually ended with the death of its host. While Chirino acknowledges that certain medical practitioners experienced some success in the treatment of the disease, there were by no means any reliable known cures. For this reason Chirino, like many of the medical writers of the time, advises that the first prophylactic step for any individual in time of pestilence should be to seek Divine intervention.

> En los tienpos de la pestilençia lo que es fazedero a los discretos omes es: Lo primero conformar con paçiençia vmilde la su boluntat con la del Señor Dios e regir sus ánimas con sanctos e claros pensamientos e con obras purgadas de todo pecado. (39)

While still offering more traditional medical advice on how to combat plague such as isolation and modified diet, Chirino is above all else a man who advocates and also actively practices a close relationship with God. Typical of the medieval man, Chirino lives in the Faith and openly admits that "Dios es la primera y última razón de todo acontecer," while still teaching therapeutic practices. A numerological study of his work shows a striking frequency of religiously charged numbers: there are three major divisions preceded by a twelve chapter section titled "reglas generales." It is not surprising, then, that the final chapter of instruction in the section on pestilence deals with a spiritual and not physical topic. Specifically, he warns against those doctors who play on a patient's fear by warning them that they could die from disease if they do not eat meat all days of the week, including Fridays. Chirino scoffs at such an absurd prognosis and warns the reader:

> el que es enemigo de la verdat non es sin razón que sea enemigo de su fija de la verdat que es la ordenança cathólica por lo qual ningunt fiel o discreto / non deue creer al médico para comer carne en viernes en ninguna enfermedat por estos temores vanos e locos juyzios. (46)

Clearly as much concerned with the spiritual as well as physical well-being of his readers, Chirino embodies the true dual nature of the medieval mind.

"Tratado útil y muy provechoso contra toda pestilencia y aire corrupto." Licenciado Fores

Written in 1481, Licenciado Fores' *Tratado vtil e muy prouechoso contra toda pestilencia e ayre corupto* offers its readers a series of preventative measures and medicinal cures specifically intended to reduce the impact of pestilence in Seville. Relatively little biographical information survives concerning Fores. María Nieves Sánchez, in a recent republication of his original manuscript, sums up what scarce data exists:

> la única fuente de datos con que contamos son las referencias académicas relativas a su vinculación con la Universidad de Salamanca. Aparece como titular de la Cátedra de Vísperas de Medicina de 1469 a 1478, aunque a partir de 1470 entra en relación con el arzobispo de Sevilla y se le sustituye en la cátedra. (7–8)

While it is fairly certain that the author lived in Seville during the writing of his work, it is unclear whether he was still alive when it was actually printed in 1507. However, despite the lack of biographical information on Licenciado Fores, it is clear from his work that he was a practitioner who was formally trained in traditional medical theory.

Typical of most of the ancient plague manuscripts, his work begins with a Latin citation from San Gregorio – this recourse to *auctoritas* is frequently employed to convey a greater authoritative tone to medical writing—and references to Galen, Avicena and Hippocrates are rather numerous as well. He is comprehensive with regard to the presentation of all known medical advice on the prevention and cure of plague and his large treatise follows a logical order. It begins with general advice on impeding the contraction of the disease and then moves on to specific information related to medicinal foods. Similar to other medical plague writers, Fores divides his treatise into two general divisions: preventative measures and cures. In the section of preventative measures, he makes further subdivisions based upon what he views as environmental or external factors (such as food, air, exercise and sleep) and internal preventative measures such as medicine. He appears to be a religious man in eloquent invocations in his Prologue and Epilogue to the Virgin Mary, Jesus and Saint Michael. However, although he shows himself to be spiritual, most of Fores' advice is firmly grounded in tangible methods for combating the disease.[22] The final result is a practical treatise that is commanding in tone and well organized in style.

Although the author originally intended his writing to address the specific instance of plague that ran unchecked throughout the city of Seville in 1481, it was actually another visitation of the disease that led to the work's publication. From 1500 to 1507, pestilential disease reoccurred in the Iberian Peninsula with a ferocity that outstripped the scourge of some twenty six years earlier.[23] Salamanca, the main educational center in the hardest hit region of Castile, published Fores' work believing that the advice contained therein would help its plague-stricken populace. Similar to Chirino, Fores' work is directed toward both "los ricos y pobres" (79) because, in his own words, "conuerna, por ello, a ser pobre, de sciencia e de cosas, no de voluntad" (80).

Always cognizant of the fact that his intended audience might not have the financial means necessary to follow properly the specifics of his medical instruction, Fores frequently offers cheaper substitutes for the ingredients that make up the medical treatments he indicates. For example, immediately following a chapter on medicinal "perfumes compuesto," he devotes another section to address "perfumes para los pobres" (86). Although he does, in fact, make similar use of juxtaposing remedies for the rich alongside those for the poor throughout the treatise, at certain points he also makes a further distinction between those who are simply poor and those who live in absolute poverty. Writing on the composition of different sorts of medicinal tonics, Fores makes suggestions for those who cannot even afford to follow his indications to "los pobres:"

> Cordial para los mas pobres
>
> Porque hay algunos tan pobres no podrian vsar destos cordiales, pueden en lo que cuezen para comer, ora sea pollo o otro manjar qualquiera, tomar vn poco de çumach e vn poco de boloarmenico quebrado vn poquillo e ponerlo en vn paño de lino delgado e muy limpio e atarlo e echarlo ansi atado a cozer con el manjar, hasta que cueza del todo el manjar (...). (149)

Such an open style of writing that has something to offer everyone from the rich to the poorest of the poor was virtually nonexistent prior to the Black Death in Europe, and its universal appeal was obviously something that seemed attractive to the Salamanca publishers of Fores' treatise.

Most of the medical advice contained in Fores' manuscript on the prevention and cure of plague is physical in nature. With preventative measures that outline everything from proper diet and grooming to the curative medical procedures that describe methods of bloodletting and mustard plasters, the information contained in the treatise follows generally accepted practical treatments of the time. On the subject of a health regimen, topics follow the order first described centuries earlier by Galen:

> (...) seys cosas son sin las quales no podemos viuir e vsando dellas como conuiene son causa de fazer sanidad, e guardarla en los cuerpos; vsando dellas en manera contraria, que es no conueniente, es causa fazedora de passion e destruydora de la sanidad. Las quales son estas: el ayre; las viandas e lo que le sigue como el beuer e medicinas; lo tercero henchimiento e su contrario; velar e dormir; exercicio o mouimiento e su contrario; las cosas que al anima acaecen como son ira, plazer, pesares. (81)

Various sections are dedicated to each of the six areas identified by Galen and special attention is given to distinguishing what to do during the hot and cold seasons. A clean house and fresh air, having now been identified as contributory factors to the propagation of disease, are strongly recommended as preventative measures while bathing, on the other hand, "se deue escusar en todas maneras, saluo los que por passiones o con consejo de medico los tomassen" (107). At the curative level, practical advice is also evidenced in the descriptions of the different levels of the disease as well as of different treatments for it. For example, one of the most detailed sections discusses where to lance an "apostema," the bubo caused by plague, depending on its location in the human body.[24] Not only does Fores quantify the amount of fluid to be drawn at "seis onzas" (122–123), he also explains the justification behind such a procedure:

> (…) porque los tales comunmente mueren con frenesis e sin juyzio o con su subeth, dormiendo; e con la sangria, si muriere, sera en su juyzio, gimiendo sus culpas e mas aliuiado de las penas del cuerpo. (126)

Avoidance of physical contact, long seen as an effective prophylactic measure, is also authoritatively spelled out in no uncertain terms.

> Escusense quanto pudieren de estar do mucha gente esta, ni en ayuntamientos, porque no sea fecha infeccion en los alientos, ca de vno se podian muchos infeccionar; deuen estar lo mas solos que puedan (…) Deuen tanbien guardarse de los que vienen de ayre inficionado y mas de los que vienen heridos (…) Avnque algun lugar este corrompido es bueno de no recebir de otro corrompido gente, especialmente si es mayor la corrupcion. El daño que oy esta en Seuilla fue por no guardar lo primero e se acrescienta por no guardar lo segundo (…). (108)

Along these same lines, he also advocates a reduction in physical contact of a sexual nature:

> El exercicio con las mugeres e llegamiento a ellas es euitar en quanto ser pueda; a lo menos, por la mayor parte, no se deuen procurar nueuas mugeres. Si algunos fueren mucho acostumbrados a ello no lo dexen del todo porque les seria dañoso; sea poco e no con mucho doñear, ca lo tal es mas enpecible; e sea hermosa e moça; deuen se apartar despues de la conuersacion dellas. (107)

However, while basing his manuscript primarily on the physical elements that man can manipulate in order to deter the lethal virus, Fores also reveals a spiritual side that creeps into his advice.

Like many medical writers of his time, he had the difficult task of trying to combine the emerging scientific data based on observation with the religious connotations traditionally associated with plague. While primarily based upon the physical steps that can be taken in order to facilitate the prevention and cure of plague, the actual advice contained within Fores' manuscript also partly attributed the onset of the disease to supernatural forces. Typical of fellow medical writers when dealing with preventative measures and cures for pestilential disease, Fores writes with an altruistic motive in order to relieve a specific outbreak in his own home town of Seville:

> (...) viendo en esta cibdad de cada dia mas nos infestar esta malicia pestilencial por nuestros pecados, con ello la absencia de los medicos, della anexa la proueza de los cibdadanos e de sus vezinos, e si los medicos avn sean tantos bien bastarian a los tales consejar, temiendo por el tal consejo auer dar dineros, como por la ignorancia de poder aprouechar remedio natural en esta passion saluo apocrifo las quales dos cosas no han lugar, por la mayor parte quise ordenar vn regimiento con alguna forma curatiua e preseruatiua breue para este morbo o passion epedimial que en estos tiempos nos cerca (...). (79–80)[25]

Connecting the outbreak to an apocalyptic punishment brought on by the sins of the citizenry of Seville, this side of Fores appears in dramatic contrast to the methodical scientist we have just discussed. However, he himself disposes of this apparent dichotomy. In the introduction to the section on cures for the pestilence, he explains that:

> (...) la diuersidad de las curas nasce de la diuersidad de las causas de las passiones, no obstante sean las tales passiones de vn mismo linage (...). (121)[26]

It is the Black Death and the new possibilities for clinical observation made possible by the vast quantities of the dead and dying that begin to call into question the older tenets, those based on divine wrath and those outdated forms of miasmatic medical theory based on equilibrium of the humors. As a result, the fourteenth and fifteenth centuries experienced new ideas on the medical nature of plague that allowed for the reconciliation of competing points of view. Specifically, new ideas with regard to etiology were typically presented alongside traditional views of miasmatic theory in order to confer greater authority to the medical writer. L. Fabian Hirst, a medical doctor tracing the evolution of epidemiology, found that authors during this time promoted their personal beliefs by stressing certain topics over others:

> It was mainly a question of the degree of emphasis to be laid upon the various factors which were believed to be in simultaneous operation, including divine power, astral influence, miasma, and contagion. (51)

This being the case, we can better understand the context under which Fores gives the following advice:

> Los feridos de la pestilencia no deuen desesperar (...) creyendo no tengan remedio; primero recorriendo a nuestro Se;or Iesuxristo, del qual procede toda medicina, como se escriue a los xxxviij capitulos del Ecclesiastico, confessando e faziendo todas las ordenanças e mandatos de la fe catholica, pues estas cosas que nos contruban e açotan las mas vezes vienen por nuestros peccados; lo segundo socorriendo nos a los remedios e beneficios [f. 11r] del arte de la medicina cuyo consejo aqui seguire (120).

An example of many similar medical texts that were produced during this period of time, the work of Licenciado Fores is important as it marks a period of transition with regard to plague theory. Once strictly believed to be brought on by supernatural forces, pestilential disease would eventually reach maturity as the more mature contagion theories developed from the eighteenth century onward.[27]

Notes

1. Translated by Ann Montgomery Campbell, *The Black Death and Men of Learning*, 52.
2. In his discussion of the Athenian plague, James Longrigg provides an excellent comparison of the manner in which Thucydides breaks with the typical Hyppocratic doctor who sacrifices accurate observation for prognosis. While such doctors would focus on theorizing the course that the disease would follow, Thucydides: "declares that his object is not to inquire into causes, but to describe the nature of the plague and set down its symptoms so that one who had foreknowledge of the disease would not fail to recognise it should it ever strike again." (31) In this manner, Thucydides makes no attempt to account for the disease in terms of the revenge of angry gods, as did his contemporaries, but rather took a more analytical and rational approach in his description.
3. Guy Beaujouan, *La Science en Espagne aux XIVe et XVe siècles* (Paris: Palais de la découverte, 1967): 7.
4. Useful studies on the six major European universities include: Pearl Kibre & Nancy Siraisi, "The Institutional Setting: Universities," in *Science in the Middle Ages*, ed. David Lindberg, (Chicago: U of Chicago P, 1978); Paul Oskar Kristeller, "School at Salerno," *Bulletin of the History of Medicine* (1945); and Anna Montgomery Campbell, *The Black Death and Men of Learning*, (New York: AMS Press, 1966): 146–180.
5. Using Ibn al-Khatib's list of fourteenth-century men of learning in the kingdom of Granada as an example, A. Campbell finds that "there are included ten physicians who died after 1347 and a monk, adept in chemistry, who seems to have exercised the functions of a physician" (95). Of these, there is evidence to show that at least three died as a direct result of contracting plague. A lack of documentation assigning the cause of death makes it difficult to establish how many of the others also died. However, if we were to apply the conclusions of Ziegler that there is no obvious reason why mortality rates would not occur in the same proportion throughout Europe (185), then the reduction of faculty members at the medical school of the University of Paris from 46 in 1348, to 26 in 1362 to 20 in 1387 shows a decidedly greater proportion of medical professionals who died or vacated their posts due to plague (Gottfried, 117).
6. By 'outside' medical practitioners, we refer to the definition as offered by Gottfried: "Structurally, the medical community was composed of five distinct

divisions: physicians, surgeons, barber-surgeons, apothecaries, and unlicensed or non professional practitioners" (104).

7. Useful works on this subject include: Carlo Cipolla, "The Professions," *The Journal of European Economic History* (1973); Thomas McKeown, *The Role of Medicine* (Princeton: Princeton UP, 1979); Vern L. Bullough, *The Development of Medicine as a Profession* (New York: Hafner, 1966); Charles H. Talbot, "Medicine," in *Science in the Middle Ages*, ed. David Lindberg (Chicago: U of Chicago P, 1978).

8. For an insightful discussion of what it meant to call oneself a surgeon rather than a physician in Spain at the beginning of the fourteenth century, see: Michael McVaugh, "Royal Surgeons and the Value of Medical Learning: the Crown of Aragon, 1300–1350," in *Practical Medicine from Salerno to the Black Death*, ed. Luís García-Ballester, et. al. (Cambridge: Cambridge UP, 1994): 211–236.

9. Luis García-Ballester, "Changes in the *Regimina sanitatis*: the Role of the Jewish Physicians," 119.

10. As was the custom of the time, the majority of the original documents transcribed and subsequently published by López de Meneses were written in Latin. As an organizational aid, López de Meneses numbered each of the 157 documents in order of what she perceived to be their date of composition but notes that some of the original manuscripts were not dated and, as such, were placed chronologically by other dated documents in the collection. To facilitate further investigations, López de Meneses also includes a brief Spanish gloss that precedes each Latin document.

11. Melanie Shirk, in her study of the work published by López de Meneses, included references to page numbers that did not correspond to the edition used in this study. For clarification, all references to López de Meneses that appeared in Shirk have been modified so as to correspond with the 1956 Zaragoza edition.

12. See Julio Valdeón, "La muerte negra en la Península," *Cuadernos de historia 16*, (Madrid: Hermanos García Noblejas, 1985): 22.

13. Shirk accurately notes that Pedro IV was surprisingly flexible in some of his approaches to solving the dilemma of administrative and legal shortages. Frequently, he increased the jurisdiction of any living official, appointed private citizens to perform administrative tasks, changed election procedures and extended terms of office. One such example can be seen in his solution to a legal dispute: "Fallecidos de la peste todos los jurisperitos de Arbucies, no hay en la villa quien resuelva los litigios surgidos y, resultando muy caros los servicios de los jueces y escribanos de Villafranca de Panadés, Pedro IV de Aragón manda al baile de Arbucies que decida las referidas cuestiones con el consejo de algún notario y de algún práctico en ellas" (No. 76).

14. In an attempt to explain the demographic system, Thomas Malthus theorized that a population will inevitably expand faster than its supply of essential natural resources needed to survive. Consequently, there would be a series of

"checks" (disease, famine, wars) that would necessarily occur to increase the death rate over the birth rate, thereby restricting overall population.

15. Of all commodity prices, the standard base of reference was wheat. According to Julio Valdeón, "En la plana de Vic el precio de la quartera de trigo pasó de cinco a quince sueldos en el periódo comprendido entre julio de 1348 y julio de 1349" (26). Although wheat prices were high in Spain before 1347, they would experience an increase that remained high until about 1375 (Herlihy, 47). Horrox recognized that, despite an increase in wages, inflation would minimize the "real-term" gain of the worker. However, the psychological effects of the rise in wages might have had the greatest effect as workers realized their new bargaining power. As a result, in the 1370s, "wages parted company with prices, and began a rise in real terms which was to continue into the fifteenth century" (Horrox, 240). For more information on the economic changes in the Crown of Aragon, see Earl J. Hamilton, *Money, Prices and Wages in Valencia, Aragon, and Navarre, 1351–1500*, Cambridge, Harvard UP, 1936.

16. It is interesting to note that in an attempt to maintain the traditional role of peasants in the feudal system, governments throughout Europe established sumptuary laws. As conspicuous consumption by the peasant—who now could afford finer foods and clothing—threatened to erase the outer signs of class distinction, laws regulating meals, fashions and customs (such as how many mourners could attend a funeral) were put into effect. Of course, sustained depopulation caused by recurrent plague epidemics kept demand for workers high thereby rendering such laws ineffective. For more information, see Herlihy, 48.

17. Such laws, or "fueros," attempted to stabilize rising prices by fixing wages as well as working conditions for almost all laborers and artisans. Specifically, regulations were put into effect that regulated the following professions: "labradores, maestros de casas, herreros, zapateros, curtidores, toneleros, cuchilleros, bataneros, sastres, pellejeros, freneros; selleros, febridores (que acicalaban las armas), escuderos, nodrizas, molineros, tejedores y notarios (Sobrequés Callicó, 73–74). Of specific interest in López de Meneses is document No. 78.

18, Charles Verlinden, *Revue belge de philologie et d'historie*, 17 (1938), 113ff., 143. For Castile see E. Mitre Fernández, *Anuario de estudios medievales*, 7 (1970–1), 615–21 (population), and J. Valdeón, *Anuario de historia económica y social*, 3 (1970), 325–35 (inflation, despite royal orders, in prices and wages).

19. It is interesting to note that Campbell sees the period of the Black Death to have been the catalyst that increased the social standing of the medical practitioner: "Till about the end of the thirteenth and the beginning of the fourteenth centuries, surgery had never been held in esteem, nor, except for a period of brilliance in Roman times, had it developed beyond a rudimentary stage. As

intellectual activity and curiosity increased in Europe, and the dependence of accurate knowledge upon experimentation became more evident, enterprising spirits began to break through tradition and prejudice." (109)

20. Unless otherwise noted, all biographical information on the life of Alonso de Chirino comes from A. González Palencia and L. Contreras Poza, *Menor daño de la medicina y Espejo de medicina*, (Madrid: Impr. de J. Cosano, 1945).

21. All references to the *Menor daño de medicina* are from the critical edition of María Teresa Herrera, Salamanca: Universidad de Salamanca, 1973. In this edition, Chirino's work is based on the Escorial manuscript published c. 1506. See Herrera XXI–XXXVIII for more information.

22. A further example that comments on both Fores' spirituality and demonstrates his outstanding organizational skills is found in his own description of his work:

> El qual tratado sera partido en dos partes principales: en regimiento preseruatiuo e la segunda curatiuo. El primero e preseruatiuo se partira en otras dos, assi que seran tres partes, a reuerencia de la Santa Trinidad. (82)

23. Carreras Panchón, 36.

24. It is noteworthy to mention that while numerous medical tractates of the time discuss buboes and the bloodletting that is their usual remedy, Fores' text is outstanding because of its detailed advice. The manuscript devotes a section to the treatment of a bubo that could possibly appear on every part of the body and even anticipates the contingency that the infected might be a female experiencing her menstrual period.

25. All references to Licenciado Fores are from his work republished by María Nieves Sánchez in *Tratados de la peste* (Madrid: Arco Libros, 1993): 77–158.

26. Fores uses the term "passiones" here as a synonym to "enfermedades."

27. For more information on the evolution of Contagion Theory, see L. Fabian Hirst: "Miasma Versus Contagion: an Historic Controversy," in *The Conquest of Plague*, (Oxford: Clarendon Press, 1953): 51–72.

• CHAPTER THREE •

Allusions to Plague: Themes in the Fictional Texts of the Iberian Peninsula

> He had come like a thief in the night. And one by one dropped the revellers in the blood-bedewed halls of their revel, and died each in the despairing posture of his fall. (Edgar Allan Poe, *The Masque of the Red Death*, 388)

It is logical to assume that a lethal disease, such as plague, combined with its widespread contamination rate and frequency of reoccurrence would have undoubtedly had a profound effect on the society in which it occurred. Having discussed the more physical aspects of the disease in our analysis of the medical documents dealing with pestilential outbreaks, we now turn to a consideration of how this calamity might have affected individual thinking. A study of the literature of the time reveals whether different works share similar underlying themes regarding plague and, if so, how do these themes represent larger ideological changes in society. Much in the same manner as Millard Meiss identified certain changes in the painting of Florence and Sienna during the time of the Black Death,[1] We highlight some literary themes common to Spanish works produced during and immediately following severe outbreaks of pestilence.

In order to guide us at this point in the study, it is important to recognize the work of two critics who have done basic groundwork in the area of analyzing "plague literature" with the goal of identifying recurrent themes in the works they consider. Both Barbara Fass Leavy's 1992 study, *To Blight with Plague*, and René Girard's 1996 publication, "The Plague in Literature and Myth," study texts of Western literature that, at first glance, appear quite diverse in terms of their subject matter.

Fass Leavy's study is comprised of various pieces of literature beginning with Giovanni Boccaccio's fourteenth-century *Decameron* and ending with AIDS-related texts of the twentieth century: Larry Kramer's *The Normal Heart* (1985); and William M. Hoffman's *As Is* (1990). Likewise, Girard also brings together works that, seemingly, would have little basis for inclusion in his study of literature related to plague. In fact, his attempt to discover certain themes related to plague literature groups together an even more diverse body of texts. For him, plague is found everywhere in literature.

> It belongs to the epic with Homer, to tragedy with *Oediups Rex*, to history with Thucydides, to the philosophical poem with Lucretius (...) the theme spans the whole range of literary and even nonliterary genres, from pure fantasy to the most positive and scientific accounts. It is older than literature—much older, really, since it is present in myth and ritual in the entire world. (155)

Since, for him, plague is everywhere in literature, his general approach is to consider diverse literary pieces such as Dostoevsky's *Crime and Punishment* and Shakespeare's *Troilus and Cressida* alongside filmwork by Ingmar Bergman as examples of works that employ the theme of plague as an underlying source of creative energy. As the apparently diverse body of works that these two critics bring together for comparison is so similar to our own study of plague-related themes in Spanish literature, a preliminary analysis of each author's findings will prove insightful for the texts we will be presenting next.

In her study, Fass Leavy's bringing together of a number of chronologically distant literary works that share the common theme of pestilent disease shows—contrary to affirmations by some previous students of plague literature who insist there is merely a linguistic similarity common to narratives which describe cities under the siege of plague—that literary works produced during or immediately following serious plague outbreaks share profound characteristics. For Fass Leavy, plague is a natural disaster whose very essence calls into question the relationship between individuals and society. As a contrast to other natural disasters such as earthquakes, floods and hurricanes, plague is an unforeseen evil that infects without reason and usually kills over a more extended period of time. In a town harshly stricken by disease, the sickness would naturally permeate the mind of all its citizens: as much the infected who are dying as the healthy who must worry about contracting the lethal affliction. With time, history tells us that the sudden shock and trauma initially generated by the onset of this biological catastrophe eventually gives way to more long-term philosophical questioning of humans and their obligations to the society in which they live.

Historically, when news spread of pestilential disease in a city, a common reaction among the fearful citizenry was to distance itself from the individuals suspected of carrying the disease. Fear of contamination, widely documented in first-hand accounts, spawned a reaction among individuals that broke down even the closest of family bonds:

> [Plague] took away all Compassion; self Preservation indeed appear'd here to be the first Law. For the Children ran away from their Parents, as they languished in the utmost Distress: And in some Places, tho' not so frequent as the other, Parents did the like to their Children (...). (Defoe, 95)

In a larger scope, the same sort of social breakdown occurred when whole families were forced into isolation from the general population in spite of the health or sickness of individual members. Pesthouses were set up and those who entered rarely exited alive. Health officials were given sweeping powers to separate the sick from the healthy so that even those who wished to care for their sick relatives were powerless to do so. Women "of honest reputation" were typically contracted to circulate through the towns in search of those who were ill. Once a victim dying of plague was discovered, governmental policy took over with unwavering resolution:

> (...) if [examiners] find any person sick of the infection, [they must] give order to the constable that the house be shut up (...) That to every infected house there be appointed two watchmen, one, for every day, and the other for the night: and that these watchmen have a special care that no person go in or out of such infected houses, whereof they have the charge, upon pain of severe punishment. (Orders Conceived and Published by the Lord Maior and Aldermen of the City of London, 197–198)[2]

Hiding a sick family member from health authorities was considered a serious crime and, consequently, severe punishments of any violations ensured the mandatory divisions between the healthy and the sick.

Unfortunately, an undesired consequence was a corresponding increase in social fissures that divided authority figures and the masses.

This public example of social breakdown, illustrated by mandatory isolation where a community openly refuses to care for its own people, is a common characteristic exemplifying social collapse at the professional level as well. Motivated by fear and the instinct for self-preservation, spiritual and physical health caregivers often shirked the social responsibilities of their vocation. As we now know after the important study of Richard Gyug, the church clergy of Spain—whose services were certainly in high demand during the Black Death—was one of the first social structures to suffer a severe breakdown. Gyug, through his research of the notarial registers of the Archivo Diocesano de Barcelona, determined that there was a dramatic increase in the rate in which beneficed clergy of this Spanish city quit their office during the years associated with plague infestations:

> Resignations (...) increase in the postplague period from an average of one every two months to about two per month.[3] (...) the doubling of duties and the increase in resignations is reinforced by a noticeable decline in revenues for the taxpaying benefices listed in *Taxae beneficiorum 1*. ("The Effects and Extent of the Black Death," 393–394)

With the risk of contamination as a result of performing various deathbed duties, many notaries, medical professionals and even members of the clergy abandoned the needs of the sick and dying. With over forty per cent of the beneficed clerics of Spain dying in the summer and fall of 1348, causing a vacancy rate some fifteen times higher than during pre-plague years, it is understandable why clerics and other professionals who had similar contact with the ill walked away from their social responsibilities.[4] Even if they had been successful in their attempt to escape contamination, such clerics and professionals undoubtedly would have provoked a great deal of both personal and public questioning through their cowardly actions. Like the parents who abandon sick children and the society that ostracizes the healthy along with the sick for its own safety, the behavior of professionals, when they abandon their social responsibilities, illustrates how plague calls into question the moral obligations of individuals within the larger society.

In Fass Leavy's finding, it is this act of questioning Man's relation to society that functions as an underlying theme of all works of literature produced during the time of virulent pestilential outbreaks. Irrespective of the diversity of their subject matter or of the era in which they were written, it is her conclusion that examples of "plague literature" all share this common trait:

> (...) despite changing conceptions of the "self," the psychological and moral issues concerning what constitutes human beings as a group and what individuates its members serve to unify works of plague literature written over centuries and within the contexts of vastly different ideas of a human relationship to the universe. (11)

Obviously, people will have differing reactions when they discover they are at risk of contracting a lethal disease. While popular reactions to a widespread pathological epidemic usually lean towards strategies of self-preservation, it would be wrong to suggest that plague automatically leads to a complete breakdown of the social contract.

To the contrary, history provides examples that demonstrate how a lethal contagion can actually lead to unexpected actions from magnanimous individuals who put themselves at risk in service of their fellow citizen. One classic example is that of Saint Roch and his legendary "miraculous powers" which he employed in the fight against the disease:

> He tirelessly tended the plague-stricken in Italian cities in the fourteenth century and was credited with many spectacular cures. But when he himself caught the disease, he was expelled from the city of Piacenza and left to die in the woods. He was saved by a nobleman's dog that daily brought him bread. Saint Roch recovered, only to die in prison in his native Montpellier, in the south of France. (Gregg, 15)

Nevertheless, though such noble actions did exist, the same basic introspection—or questioning of the individual and his relationship with society—comes into play. "Just as illness in an individual forces the relaxation of social and moral attitudes," writes David Steel, "so disease on a vast social scale liberates cynicism and lawlessness" (90). It is precisely this relaxation of social and moral attitudes that brings about the introspection of which we speak. It also frames the impetus behind the "thematic clusters" that Girard considers a universal characteristic of plague literature.[5]

In "The Plague in Literature and Myth," Girard affirms that all forms of plague in imaginative writing are similar to one another despite the thematic and, often, temporal distance that separates them. Comparing a diverse body of plague writing that spans the centuries from Thucydides to Camus, Girard affirms that:

> (...) there is a strange uniformity to the various treatments of the plague, not only literary and mythical but also scientific and non-scientific, of both past and present. Between the matter-of-fact, even statistical account of Defoe in his *Journal of the Plague Year* and the near hysteria of Artoud in *Le Théâtre et la peste*, the differences, at close range, turn out to be minor. (155)

For Girard, the many forms of plague writing are unquestionably bound together in the manner through which they all explore the notion of the similar. In this respect, the differences that exist between various examples of plague writing over time and space are of a truly superficial nature. The essence of such texts is that they, like plague in general, are based on "a process of undifferentiation, a destruction of specificities" (Girard, 155). Just as we have seen in our study of the medical tractates that document various reactions to pestilential outbreaks, this destruction of the specificities of which Girard speaks is often preceded by a reversal of both a monetary and social ethos:

> The plague will turn the honest man into a thief, the virtuous man into a lecher, the prostitute into a saint. Friends murder and enemies embrace. Wealthy men are made poor by the ruin of their business. Riches are showered upon paupers who inherit in a few days the fortunes of many distant relatives. Social hierarchies are first transgressed, then abolished. Political and religious authorities collapse. The plague makes all accumulated knowledge and all categories of judgement invalid. (155)

Pestilential disease, in contrast with other kinds of natural disasters, stands apart, unique in that it temporarily does away with all forms of social distinction.

Indeed, social boundaries are one of the first frontiers breached in any serious outbreak of plague. It is precisely for this reason that Camus emphatically focuses on this point throughout his fiction, *The Plague*. After many weeks of imposed isolation in the shut-off city of Oran, the citizens are described as a single entity brought together by their shared experiences:

> No longer were there individual destinies; only a collective destiny, made of plague and the emotions shared by all. Strongest of these emotions was the sense of exile and of deprivation, with all the cross-currents of revolt and fear set up by these. (157)

The disease itself also effectively breaks down individual boundaries owing to its particular pathology of killing the young as readily as the old, the rich as well as the poor. As we previously noted in our discussion of Spanish historical documents dealing with plague, the disease also generates the redistribution of wealth, usually bettering the economic standings of the poor at the expense of the rich. Accordingly, most written documents produced around the times of virulent plague epidemics commonly show an increase in themes that center upon this idea of a "destruction of specificities" of individuals within a society. This is a common feature of plague literature written in many lands over centuries and is clearly also represented in the works of medieval Spain.

As we will present in a future section of this study, the most obvious Spanish example of this great leveling of members of society is the late fourteenth to early fifteenth-century *Dança general de la Muerte*. Gradually progressing from king to cleric to peasant, the underlying message is unmistakable: in spite of one's social status in life, the vanities of this world will quickly be forgotten as the final dance with Death fulfills its function as the great equalizer. However, while this particular literary example may seem obvious, since many variations on the Dance of Death theme produced in times of plague are abundant throughout Europe, Girard takes this theory one step further in his explanation of works that he considers examples of plague literature. In his view, this theme of *undifferentiation* of members in a society is but one small sub-category of what he refers to as a larger "thematic cluster" of plague literature.

Girard believes—despite the diverse nature of their topics—all works of plague literature revolve around a nuclear thematic cluster rather than one specific theme. In his words, this thematic cluster includes "...besides the plague or, more generally, the theme of epidemic contamination, the dissolving of differences and the mimetic *doubles*" (162). Citing examples from Shakespeare and Dostoevsky, he goes on to affirm that this thematic cluster:

> (...) almost never fails to gather around the plague in a great many texts that may appear to have very little in common. Some of the elements may be

more emphasized than others; they may appear only in an embryonic form, but it is very rare when even one of them is completely missing. (162)

In addition to the aforementioned elements, Girard names one last—not insignificant—component of this thematic cluster: the *sacrificial* element. In this critic's view, the death and suffering resulting from plague is a process necessary for the eventual purification and rejuvenation of a society. Death, in many texts written during the time of plague outbreaks, leads readers to question their own existence by taking on – or identifying with—a central role in a story's main argument. In this sense, the idea of death serving as a cleansing element is closely linked to the idea of the scapegoat:

> Death itself appears as the purifying agent, the death of all plague victims or a few, sometimes of a single chosen victim who seems to assume the plague in its entirety and whose death or expulsion cures the society, in the rituals of much of the world. Sacrifices and the so-called scapegoat rituals are prescribed when a community is stricken by "the plague" or other scourges. (163)

Much in the same way that Jewish civilians were often accused of bringing on the plague by poisoning wells throughout Spain, the scapegoat figure—individual or collective—served the purposes of unifying a fragmented society during the times of pestilential outbreaks.[6]

As the act of striking out against those who appeared to be "outsiders" to a given society would also inherently put distance between the object of hatred and the aggressor, one can claim that it is hubristic pride and the desire to differentiate oneself from the victims that resulted in overt violence. However, this same logic can hold true with relation to the social breakdowns mentioned earlier. When father disowns son and societies ostracize entire families in the name of protecting themselves from the plague, they are, in a real sense, also offering members of its societies as sacrificial victims. Hubristic pride is also at work here for the healthy citizens implicitly attempt to differentiate themselves from the afflicted by professing a certain mastery over that mysterious piece of information—be it a more resistant physical makeup at the physical level or a greater degree of spirituality on the metaphysical side—that eluded those unfortunates stricken with the disease.

It is Girard's opinion that all the thematic elements of this cluster are juxtaposed in plague literature itself and that their presence need not be accompanied by explicit references to plague. In fact, it is in the *Scapegoat* that this critic first presents the argument that there was actually an effort made by authors to *avoid* direct references to plague.[7] Offering Guillaume de Machaut's mid-fourteenth century poem *Judgment of the King of Navarre* as a source, Girard argues:

> Medieval communities were so afraid of the plague that the word alone was enough to frighten them. They avoided mentioning it as long as possible and even avoided taking the necessary precautions at the risk of aggravating the effects of the epidemic. So helpless were they that telling the truth did not mean facing the situation but rather giving in to its destructive consequences and relinquishing all semblance of normal life. The entire population shared in this type of blindness. (2–3)

However, despite the superstitious avoidance of the term 'plague'—for fear of facing the reality of its unbridled destructive force—the idea of plague and its devastating effects can be seen in other ways. Because the extreme disruption caused by the epidemic undermined social cohesiveness and order, one result was a challenge to society's traditional religious, political and philosophical underpinnings. Girard argues that, because the disease involves both personal physical and collective emotional deterioration, the literature produced in and around the years of pestilential outbreaks best reflects the cultural sentiment of the time. Perhaps, then, in the crucible of the heightened awareness of a writer's sensibilities, their craft becomes the best gauge of changes in the cultural imagination. As we shall see, the literature produced in the time of plague in Spain does indeed suffer a notable transformation and that this change involves the basic ideological tenants of Man's perceptions of death and dying. However, it is also important to recognize that such novel visions do not necessarily depend on direct representation.

As seen in the discussion of ancient works on plague, the term "plague" had from the beginning a notoriously vague meaning and has been associated with the definition of a specific disease only in recent years.[8] For this reason, the Spanish medical writers previously discussed often resorted to citing both physical and metaphysical reasons for the visitation of the disease when faced with having to explain authoritatively the cause and prevention of an infirmity that they themselves did not fully understand. For them, as well as for the writer of fiction of the time, the key to comprehending the unexpected reoccurrence of plague in their society was based on the concept of order. Disturbances in cosmological forces, the natural balance of the four humors or the balance between the body and the soul were all viewed as pre-conditions that could bring about the onset of pathological epidemics. Such imbalances, if not corrected through proper identification and intervention by the medical or spiritual authorities, only could end in death.

For this reason, medical writers often used a combination of both physical cures—such as phlebotomy—in conjunction with metaphysical remedies—such as advising patients to pay greater attention to their Biblical Commandments. Obviously, their conception of the term "plague" referred to both the physical symptoms that afflicted an individual as well as to the unseen, or more metaphysical, disturbance in the universe leading to such an infirmity. Thus, competent medics typically needed to address both possible sources of the disease in their diagnoses. Despite how irrational this concept may appear today, the interrelationship between the physical and metaphysical universe had ancient origins and was still widely accepted in the Middle Ages:

> Earlier physicians like Galen regarded Nature, which formed the body, as a divine instrument. The moral tradition taught that the body housed the soul; both should work harmoniously as part of a larger, divine plan. Writers who held a moral view believed that plague resulted from poor governance of both soul and body. (Stieve, 236)

Thus, educated medical writers typically included both physical and metaphysical elements in their discourse on the plague. However, it is also clear that this form of science-oriented writing tended to favor the more physical aspects of prevention and cure of the disease. The writer of fiction, on the other hand, was lacking in medical training and sought to explain the visitation through expression of the imagination. While still keeping in step with the concept of plague resulting from a disturbance in the natural "order" of things, fiction writers who compose in the heart and in the aftermath of serious plague epidemics tend to emphasize the more intangible, spiritual causes of the outbreak. Taking advantage of the social desperation that repeated outbreaks of disease provoked in the citizenry, post-Black Death writing of a fictional nature in Spain sought to use imagery of death and disease in somewhat original ways. Above all else, this addition to plague literature emphasizes the graphic characteristics of plague: the putrefying corpse, the gross exaggeration of the literal and the anthropomorphic figure of death as means for examining some greater moral issues.

As noted, part of the ease of overlooking the impact of recurrent plague epidemics on the literature of Spain is that there are, in fact, relatively few explicit textual references to the calamity during the years in question. While medical texts, demographic studies and historical documents all verify that this contagious lethal infection was widespread in the Iberian Peninsula, imaginative texts only rarely focus *specifically* on this topic. Instead, fictional writing at this time frequently shows an increased attraction to other topics that involve the subject of death and corporal decay. Obviously, the growth in morbid fascination with the grossly literal comes as a result of the frequency with which everyday citizens came into contact with the dead and the dying. Plague, according to eyewitnesses, is nightmarish in its pathology and causes physical deformations that offend both the sight and smell of those surrounding the victim. Referring to a plague outbreak in 1665, Thomas Vincent describes the effects of the disease in the following manner:

> It is so poysonous a disease; it poysons the blood and the spirits, breeds a strange kind of venom in the body, which breaketh forth sometimes in Boils and Blains, and great Carbuncles (...) it turns the good humors into putrefaction, which putting forth it self in the issues of running sores, doth give a most noysome smell. (from *God's Terrible Voice in the City* published in 1667)[9]

Likewise, in *A Journal of the Plague Year*, Daniel Defoe confirms that plague is widespread by nature and attacks nearly every household with unwavering ferocity once it enters a city:

> (...) the prodigious Number that were taken sick the Week or two before, besides those that dies, was such, and the Lamentations were so great every where, that a Man must have seemed to have acted even against his Reason, if he had so much as expected to escape; and as there was hardly a House, but mine, in all my Neighborhood, but what was infected. (191)[10]

However, while this increase in the contact that citizens of all social classes in Spain and throughout Europe had with horrific scenes of death and dying was a contributory element in the increase of fictional writings that centered on physical decay, in light of the arguments of Fass Leavy, Steele and Girard, it is more likely that this new fascination was inspired by changing metaphysical ideologies. Instead of simply employing morbid imagery for its shock value, for an audience that certainly had increased sensitivities with respect to the subject, the interest in this new theme reflects deep-rooted changes regarding medieval attitudes towards human mortality.

For centuries, the Church had depicted physical death as a natural, even a blessed, transition from this world to the next. Rituals, being a religious tool to help ease the pain of losing a loved one, helped console the living as much as it purported to help the dead achieve eternal rest. Separation, then, was only temporary as the living would one day be reunited with the dead through their own passing. Such death rituals provided the balm which helped restore order:

> The rituals thus encouraged the living to accept the lost of their loved ones, recruit others to continue the work of the departed, mend the rift in the social fabric that death had caused, and return now to their quotidian labors. Through these rites of passage, not only the dead but the living too were introduced into a new phase of existence. (Herlihy, 60)

The onset of lethal plague pandemics, however, changed all this. Gyug was one of the first critics to comment on how the ecclesiastical records of Barcelona reveal a chaos, owing to plague outbreaks, among the religious orders that likely mirrored reactions throughout the peninsula. His first observation is that the turnover rate in professional clergymen forced the scribes to adopt a new condensed way of formally documenting such changes.

> Instead of notice of a presentation and copies of two letters, one for appointment, the other for execution, most cases are treated in a single highly abbreviated entry (…) the document [was] no longer a complete transcript but rather a précis of an entire series of official letters. (…) The business of providing for vacant benefices so overwhelmed the diocesan administration that not only were documents noted in a more cursory fashion but the amount of other business was sharply limited. ("Effects and Extent," 392–394)

The reasons for such abridged versions are obvious. When during normal months a scribe would typically have to produce slightly over eight documents per month, during plague-related months this number grew to an astounding fifty-eight per month.[11] Likewise, he notes that such documents concerning the mitigation of problems due to vacant churches also suggest turmoil among the religious leaders of the community.

> A category of documents which appears for the first time in *Notule communium* 15 allowed the temporary appointment of already beneficed clergy to the care of souls and the collection of tithes in churches that had lacked rectors for some time. (...) The need to shift duties onto someone already beneficed implies either that the number of eligible candidates was limited or that diminished congregations neither required nor could support full-time rectors. (Gyug, 393)

With the decrease in active clergy owing to flight or death, burial practices necessarily had to be adjusted to deal with the consistently high mortality rates. Extreme Unction, or the last anointing in which the dying make a bedside confession of sin to their priest, quickly evolved from being, typically, a private affair to becoming a mass public ceremony or, in a few cases, unavailable altogether. Boccaccio, describing consequences of the Black Death in Florence, paints a grim scene that portrays vividly the increased pressures put upon clergymen in times of pestilential outbreak:

> And times without number it happened that two priests would be on their way to bury someone, holding a cross before them, only to find that bearers carrying three or four additional biers would fall in behind them; so that whereas the priests had thought they had only one burial to attend to, they in fact had six or seven, and sometimes more. Even in these circumstances, however, there were no tears or candles or mourners to honour the dead; in fact, no more respect was accorded to dead people than would nowadays be shown towards dead goats. (*Decameron*, 56)

Given the demographic evidence of plague in the Iberian Peninsula, this scene assuredly would have played out in a similar manner in Spain. Thus, with such inevitable shortcomings of the clergy regarding the spiritual well-being of their congregations, it is hardly surprising that perceptions of death changed. No longer was human mortality viewed as a benign natural process of transition, rather death was now *seen* as a horrible and violent Enemy of Man. As an imaginary representation of this newly forged, negative perception of human mortality, the image of the putrefying corpse and the stark personification of Death took center-stage.

In order better to understand the meaning behind the literary use of images such as the putrefying corpse and Death personified as implacable, one needs to be familiar with the general function of symbols in the Middle Ages for, as an effective tool for conveying ideas to an illiterate populace, the evocation of ideas through symbols was common. Symbolism, and the numerous connotations we still associate with it, often derive meaning from the traditions of the pagan or Christian societies of antiquity. According to Ladner, the founding Fathers of the Church used the term 'symbol' in two distinct manners:

> They spoke of a Symbol of the Christian Faith, by which they meant the Creed. It was a 'drawing together,' a summary and token, of the main truths and doctrines of Christianity (...) The second meaning of symbol that was current in early Christian times (...) is very close to, or even synonymous with, *semeion, signum,* sign—Origin says that whatever happens in an unexpected or strange way in Holy Scripture is a 'semeion kai symbolon,' a sign or symbol, of something else, namely of something beyond the realm of sense experience. (224)

To the religious leaders of the community, official Church doctrine was ineffable by nature and, therefore, needed to be conveyed by use of images. In this manner, the "unopened vessel" came to represent the Virgin Mary, jeweled crosses became the symbol of the transfigured Christ and the Byzantine basilica and later Christian cathedrals imitated Man's conception of Heavenly Paradise.[12] As religious thought became more sophisticated with time, so the development of associated imagery became more complex.

The need for conveying abstract religious thought by way of tangible associations eventually led to an over abundance of sacred images. In the fourteenth century, for example,

> (...) the cross and the lamb no longer sufficed for the effusions of overflowing love offered to Jesus; to these is added the adoration of the name of Jesus (...) Henry Suso tattoos the name of Jesus over his heart and compares himself to the lover who wears the name of his beloved embroidered on his coat. Bernardino of Siena, at the end of a moving

sermon, lights two candles and shows the multitude a board a yard in length, bearing on an azure ground the name Jesus in golden letters, surrounded by the sun's rays. (Huizinga, 200)

With time the religious concept and the symbolic representation that referred to it became so thoroughly assimilated in the mind of Medieval man that the symbol often grew to the point of replacing the original idea that spawned it.

> The mere presence of a visible image of things wholly sufficed to establish their truth. No doubts intervened between the sight of all those pictures and statues—the persons of the Trinity, the flames of hell, the innumerable saints—and the belief in their reality. All these conceptions became matters of faith in the most direct manner; they passed straight from the state of images to that of convictions, taking root in the mind as pictures clearly outlined and vividly coloured, possessing all the reality claimed for them by the Church, and even a little more. (Huizinga, 165).

So powerful was this use of symbolic imagery that it eventually passed from depicting purely religious concepts to wider uses delving into profane and moral topics. As an effective form of artistic expression, it is no surprise that literature comes to be a powerful example of this evolution. Wholly symbolic in nature and powerful in its ability to play to the five senses of its audience, the fiction in the years surrounding disease outbreaks show the greatest sophistication in the detailed concept of physical decay and the use of the putrefying corpse. Beginning around the mid-fourteenth century in the Iberian Peninsula, this movement that swept Europe is a direct reflection of man's changing attitudes as a result of plague.

Libro de (la) miseria d'omne

Little is known about the 502 strophe work that we typically refer to as the *Libro de miseria d'omne*. Ian Michael, one scholar who has studied the poem, offers a succinct overview of the existing data we have on the verse that most researchers believe was composed around the year 1375.[13]

> The *Libro de miseria de omne* is a *cuaderna vía* poem dating ... from the end of the century. The manuscript was found in a ruined tower in a village in La

> Montaña (prov. of Santander) in 1919. This pessimistic work is based on a famous treatise by Pope Innocent III, *De contemptu mundi*. It deals with the miseries of mankind, and includes some satirical comments on contemporary society. (227)

To critics such as Alan Deyermond, the *Libro de miseria* is interesting not only at the thematic level—attributable to its gloomy warnings against the miseries of mortal life, the sins of the individual and the evils of the world,—but also because it possesses an arresting technical deviation. Along with such poems as the irregular *Proverbios de Salmón*,[14] the *Libro de miseria* strays from the standard *cuaderna vía* verse form that was the dominant Castilian literary form of the first half of the thirteenth century. Deyermond describes this deviation in the following terms:

> The versification has one unusual feature: instead of the fourteen-syllable line normal in *cuaderna vía*, the poet consistently uses lines of sixteen, divided into two hemistichs. This may well show the influence of the ballad line (...) which consists of eight-syllable hemistichs; but if so, the poem must have been compposed towards the end of the century (*The Middle Ages*, 108)

Taken in conjunction with works such as the *Doctrina de la discriçión* (also known as the *Tractado de la doctrina*), Deyermond argues the *Libro de miseria* is especially important as a representative of what he calls a departure from the standard form fomented by the monastic school of *clerecía* poets. However, apart from being considered on its technical form, the *Libro de miseria d'omne* is also interesting at the thematic level for the manner in which it employs lugubrious images to rivet the attention of its intended audience at the individual level. Despite the fact that it was actually based on another literary work that predates the first known occurrence of medieval plague in the Iberian Peninsula, the *Libro de miseria d'omne* is interesting precisely for the new contextualization it adopts in adapting Innocent III's original work. With the implicit purpose of reaching out to a contemporary audience in a direct, stark and persuasive manner, the anonymous author of the *Libro de miseria d'omne* employs the use of graphic and grotesque imagery as a means to illustrate an urgent didactic message. Above all else, this didactic message centers on the topic of moral disorder and how this chaos is evident at all levels of late fourteenth-century Iberian society.

• CHAPTER THREE •

Jane E. Connolly is the most important scholar to recognize that, although the anonymous poet of the *Libro de miseria d'omne* declared the source of his work to be the late twelfth-century treatise *De miseria condicionis humane*, the innovations introduced into the later work make it a imaginative example of independent thinking. In Connolly's opinion, the current lack of critical interest in the *Libro de miseria* is an unfortunate result of previous scholars' inability to see the work as anything but a simple translation of a Latin original. She accurately identifies the error of such a classification:

> I believe the term "translation" falls into this category of the imprecise and inconsistent, and the fact that the word frequently appears enclosed in quotation marks or accompanied by qualifying explanations seems to describe the relationship of the *Libro de miseria* to the *De Miseria*, for it conveys the idea of transmitting the Latin text rather than transforming it. When considering works such as the *Libro de miseria*, we would be better to restrict ourselves to terms such as poet/poem rather than translator/ translation, for the author does not blindly follow the source but rather adapts and recreates it to meet his own artistic and personal designs. (49)

In the same manner that Brian Dutton's numerous studies of the relationship of Berceo's poems to their original sources prove that the latter poet uses his own sources to produce his own independent creative works,[15] one can clearly see that the omissions and expansions of the author of the *Libro de miseria* establish that this poem is, indeed, an independent creative work. Bearing in mind that this poem was produced during the time of an exceptionally virulent plague outbreak, it is precisely these changes and omissions that interest us.

In his study of Juan Ruiz's *Libro de buen amor*, Manuel Criado de Val argued that the work itself—and, specifically, the large passage on Doña Endrina—was often dismissed by scholars as an example of imaginative Spanish medieval writing only because it was based on an earlier prototype.

> El largo pasaje de <<Doña Endrina>> ha sido en muchas ocasiones desvalorizado, torpemente por considerarlo una simple paráfrasis de un viejo texto latino medieval, el *Pamphilus de amore*. No es fácil explicar cómo un aprendiz puede superar tan radicalmente a su supuesto maestro, aunque es evidente que Juan Ruiz sigue paso a paso la intriga amorosa del texto latino. Comparar <<Doña Endrina>> con el <<Pamphilus>> es un magnífico

ejercicio de análisis estilístico; una muestra del propósito <<recreativo>> que define a un gran número de obras medievales. (185)

Although he speaks only of the *Libro de buen amor*, Criado de Val's argument could easily be applied to the *Libro de miseria d'omne*; the later work, took is a valid "ejercicio de análisis estilístico; una muestra del propósito <<recreativo>> (...)." Connolly adds,

> Since the publication of Miguel Artigas' paleographic edition of the *Libro de miseria de omne*, (...) there has been little study of the poem. Indeed this work has been relegated to the remote corners of our literary histories, if it appears in them at all. (...) Hispanists who have considered the *Libro de miseria* have focused their attention on two interrelated aspects: (1) the date of composition and (2) the poem as a manifestation of the decay of the *quaderna vía*. The results of their examinations are inconclusive and often misleading. (Connolly, i)

Summarily dismissed by scholars such as Ricardo Ciérvide, Dámaso Alonso, Francisco López Estrada and Rosa Boba Naves for its perceived lack of literary value, the *Libro de miseria* has been unfairly neglected.[16] However, when considered alongside its original Latin ancestor, the anonymous Spanish poem reveals itself to be not only an interesting independent form of artistic expression but also a good representative of the literature produced in the wake of plague pandemics.

As previously noted, Connolly is one of the first scholars to recognize the importance of comparing the *Libro de miseria* to its original Latin source as this was the best way to discern the true creative force (content and style) of the Spanish poem. In an attempt to resolve the issue of its originality, she examined the relationship between the two works in great detail and published her findings as supplementary material to her 1987 edition of the *Libro de miseria*. As the focus of this study hopes to shed light on how the medical and imaginary literature could have been affected by medieval plague—and not the specific differences between the *Libro de miseria* and its Latin prototype—we can use the conclusions of Connolly's findings to substantiate our own claims.

One of the first matters to catch Connolly's eye in her deft comparison of the two poems is the obvious difference in the language in which each author composes his work. However, while one would expect appropriate linguistic changes to occur when translating a document from one language to another, Connolly's examination concludes that the Spanish poet makes substantial stylistic changes to the Latin original. It has been argued that Innocent's *De Miseria* was originally composed in a cold and austere rhetorical style.

> Most modern scholars who have studied Innocent's work have insisted primarily on the widespread influence of the *De Miseria*;[17] nonetheless, many critics have pronounced a negative judgement concerning the style of the treatise. For example, Achille Luchaire, one of the principal biographers of Innocent, labels the *De Miseria* an "exercise d'écolier, thèse de théoricien frais émolu de la scolastique."[18] Antonio Viscardi declares that Innocent writes "con la pacatezza del retore, con la sicura freddezza dello scienziato," and says that his language is "freddo e studiato—se non proprio impacciato e artificioso—e compostamente oratorio."[19] Such assessments of the *De Miseria* are unfair, for they evaluate the work according to modern standards rather than judging it from the perspective of Innocent's contemporaries. What strikes us as a coldly rhetorical and artificial style was considered to be the norm. What we view as being negative characteristics in the *De Miseria* are qualities that were expected and admired by Innocent's learnèd readers. (2–3)

In contrast, the anonymous poet of the *Libro de miseria* declares that he will not only translate the Latin original into Spanish but also offers insight into his motivation for the transformations he will incorporate. From the opening lines of the poem, we learn:

> Libro de miseria d'omne   sepades que es llamado;
> compuso esas razones   en buen latín esmerado;
> no lo entiende tod omne,   si non el que es letrado,
> por que yaze oy de muchos   postpuesto e olvidado (3)[20]

Similar to what we saw in the plague writing of a strictly medical nature, the author of the Spanish poem shows concern for reaching the understanding of the most common members of his intended audience. Not only does the poet adopt the familiar form of the *cuaderna vía*, but he also transforms the elevated and elaborate style of the Latin original into something more colloquial. Unlike his predecessor, the anonymous author writes for an audience of heterogeneous citizens and, with this in mind, he modifies the original Latin text in such a way so as to assure that his message would be easily understood by even the simplest member of his audience. Unmistakable in this attention to its intended audience, the *Libro de miseria* is not a simple translation but, rather, is a complex recreation of a work designed to meet specific artistic and didactic goals, and to address contemporary realities.

Connolly's second conclusion when comparing the *Libro de miseria* with its Latin predecessor is that the changes found in the later work indicate that its author was fundamentally concerned with producing a work that was much clearer and more coherently-structured than the original.

> Throughout his adaptation of the Latin material, the poet observes the rule of rhetorical simplicity. As we have seen, he reduces or eliminates most forms of ornamentation found in the *De Miseria* (the various types of accumulation, complex sentence structures, wordplay, etc.), employing the simple but descriptive language prescribed by St. Francis (...) we find this desire for clarity manifested primarily in the poet's tendency to explain the meaning of his material and to give advice. It is further seen in his desire to establish logical connections between each section by means of transitions, summaries and the reorganization of the Latin source. Moreover, a wish for clarity may be observed in the poet's transformation of the Latin ambiguity or abstractness, for he frequently substitutes the concrete for the abstruse by using specific *exempla*. Quite often, these *exempla* are taken from contemporary life, a practice common to mendicant preachers (...). (44–45)

Keeping in mind the tumultuous time period in which it was written (c. 1375), it is not surprising that the *Libro de miseria* substantially deviates from the Latin original with much added graphic and macabre imagery, providing the means to hone the specific messages impress upon his public. For example, the title of the third book, "*De* la podredumbre *de* las carnes," sets the macabre tone for the entire section to follow. Above all, this section in particular stresses the implicit, inverse connection between earthly pleasures and physical corruption.

> Quando el alma mesquina
> non sabe el algariva
> mas la carne malfadada
> ca tornar abrá en polvo
>
> del cuerpo ha de salir,
> a quál parte ha de ir,
> esto non podrá foír
> e en tierra de podrir.
>
> Demás quanto él ganare
> fasta'l día que moriere,
> si non fuere oración
> no levará otra cosa
>
> del día que fue nacido
> todo non vale un figo,
> o buenas obras que fizo,
> de quanto ganó consigo.
>
> (431–432)

As if to evoke the horrors of a sentient being experiencing its own slow putrefaction, the anonymous poet openly warns his intended audience to conduct themselves in a manner which honors their Christian faith. It is only through strict adherence to religious doctrines—refraining from evil and striving to lead a good life—that one might avoid the torment of Hell and gain eternal salvation.

Later, physical corruption is used as a means by which to foreground again the poet's underlying didactic messages.

> Quando es bivo el omne,   cría mota sin mesura
> de piojos e lombrizes   ca tal es la su natura;
> muerto, cría los gujanos   con su mala podredura
> que lo roen e lo comen,   dentro en su sepultura.
>
> Quando es bivo el omne,   da fructos de mal sabor,
> e desend quando es muerto, podredura e fedor;
> ond non es cosa 'nel mundo que omne quiera peor
> que tener muerto en casa   maguer aya grand dolor.
>
> (435–436)

Once again equating the vivid depiction of physical corruption after death with man's propensity to act in sinful manners in life, our poet encourages repentance and abstention from vice. The use of such graphic and grotesque imagery would have made an instant connection with an intended audience that suffered from over exposure to plague related deaths. As a means of establishing clear illustrations to underlying didactic messages, then, an increase in the use of such imagery corresponds, logically, to the omnipresence of the author's experience of surrounding pestilent epidemics.

Connolly's final observation in her comparison of the *Libro de miseria* to its Latin predecessor is that the former is fundamentally different from its source in its didactic frame. With regard to the *De Miseria*, it is clear from its highly rhetorical style, use of lofty language and haphazard presentation of standard religious topics that Innocent III's work was an expository treatment of Christian doctrine that was intended for a highly learnèd audience. As such, the examination of his topics are often characterized by needless duplicative detail or ill-developed broad generalities. In contrast, the *Libro de miseria* characteristically eliminates the repetitive quotations found in the original in order better to develop the basic ideas that remain. For example, in a style that appears frequently in many passages throughout the *De Miseria*, the section that discusses the many vices of Man results in an impersonal and superficial listing of the different types of sinners. The Spanish version, in comparison, is markedly different, as Connolly's study clarifies.

> While the Latin passage is merely a summary of sins, the Spanish passage constitutes an unmitigated attack on every level of society in which no class or office is spared. The scope of our poet's invective is quite impressive and comprehensive: *clérigo, beneficiado, prelado, sacerdote, cavallero, escudero, mercador, buhón, panadera, pescador, cavador, molinero, çapatero, ferrero, carniciero, tafur, servienta, serviente, pastor, carpentero, labrador*. No one escapes the poet's scathing criticism (...). (38–39)

Similar to what we will find in later works such as the *Dança general de la Muerte* as well as in the *Rimado de palacio* and the *Libro de Alexandre*, this sort of social criticism that speaks in concrete terms of every day abuses is something that is altogether missing in the earlier Latin work. Undoubtedly, the author of the *Libro de miseria* constructed his work with the intention of providing clear religious instruction to a vast and primarily uneducated audience. His focus on the physical decay of the human body after death—itself evoking images of a greater corruption of this world as a whole due to the sinful nature of Man—is the means by which he hopes to lead his intended reader to conduct themselves in a manner befitting eternal salvation. Keeping in mind the words of Jauss who argues that every form of medieval literature has its own "locus in life," determined by the work's historical setting and intended audience, it is not surprising that this class of writing appears at this specific point in time.[21] Reflecting both the pessimism as well as the perceived social disorder of its environment, the *Libro de miseria* and its gloomy warning of the miseries of life is a good example of literature showing strong plague influences.

Revelaçión de un hermitanno

The *Revelaçión de un hermitanno* is a short poetic work that represents a renewal of interest in the debate-poems that was current in Spain around the end of the fourteenth century.[22] Taking as its immediate model the Latin Visio Philiberti,[23] this anonymous 25 stanza poem produced c. 1382 in Spain follows a long tradition of similar debate-poems that all share similar characteristics.[24] Although poems of this type can be found in Arabic and Hebrew, the principal ancestral roots of such works derive from ninth century European origins. Typically written in Latin for a learnèd audience, the earliest debate-poems—such as the thirteenth century Altercatio Yemis et Estatis and the Conflictus Veris et Hiemis—commonly dramatize a clash between two (or sometimes more) points of view on a central issue.[25] As Deyermond has shown, the central issues of such early works usually were in direct relation to urgent issues of the era in which they were first circulated.

> A wide variety of topics is covered: theological (body and soul, Christianity and Judaism); social (knight's mistress and clerk's mistress, friar and layman, priests and peasants); erotic (love and an old man, heterosexual and homosexual love); philosophical (Fortune and the philosopher); economic (both theoretical, as in the debate between expansionists and restrictionist economics, and clashes of veested interests: wool and flax, wine and beer).
> (*Literary History*, 72)

As an example of a debate-poem that adopts an urgent contemporary issue as a central theme, the *Revelación de un hermitanno* is a fine specimen. Thematically based on an intricate body/soul debate in which each entity is represented as an independent animate object engaging in fierce accusations of one another for causing their eternal damnation, their hatred for one another is established from the very beginning. The Cuerpo, initially presented as an object of "chico balor" with a putrid smell and horrific appearance, is immediately harangued by the Alma which attacks as if it were a wild animal with "bos aguda muy fierra" (st. 3). Despite the expectations that there will be a clear winner in their battle—the Ánima, for example, proving it had been innocently betrayed by the savage Cuerpo—such a resolution never occurs. By the end of their short debate, the Cuerpo convincingly proves that the Ánima was equally to blame for any wrongdoings in life claiming that "mis pies y manos por ty [el Ánima] se mouieron" and that the ultimate findings of guilt would be in the hands of God: "pues el sennor nos ha de jusgar." (st. 8; 11). As a good representative of plague literature, this outcome is especially important as it exemplifies Girard's "destruction of specificities" previously discussed at the beginning of this chapter. Taking this element into account alongside the frequent tendencies of depicting the grossly literal by way of physical decomposition, the grim vision of the *Revelaçión de un hermitanno* can be viewed as a direct result of the psychological impact of plague.

Written in the elevated style of *arte mayor*—a poetic form that we see also in the *Dança general de la Muerte*—the *Revelaçión de un hermitanno* narrates the life of a saintly hermit who experiences a revelation in the early morning after a night engrossed in deep religious contemplation. After a brief introductory stanza which serves to establish the background of the hermit/speaker, he begins the narration of his dream vision. Immediately, the description sets the dark and somber tone that will carry on throughout the work.

> En vn balle fondo, escuro, apartado,
> Espeso de xaras, sonné que andaua
> Buscando salida e non la fallaua, (st. 2)[26]

This initial setting of a dark, distant and foreign valley is quite in step with what Susan Sontag identifies as a metaphorical connection to physical illness. As she concludes, "there is a link between imagining disease and imagining foreignness" (136). The strange foreign land is regarded, at least potentially, as a source of pollution from which one is unable to escape. Once established, this initial gloomy confusion quickly gives way to the first encounter with and subsequent graphic presentation of the corpse.

> Topé con un omne que yasia fynado.
> Holia muy mal, ca estaua fynchado,
> Los ojos quebrados, la fas denegrida,
> La boca abierta, la barga cayda,
> De gusanos e moscas muy acompannado. (st. 2)

The physical deterioration of the Cuerpo is described in ways that repulse at both the physical and olfactory levels. The blackened face is grotesquely decayed and worm-ridden while the telltale malodorous smells denote a highly advanced state of decomposition. The body is soon approached and berated by its own soul taking the shape of a white bird "batiendo las alas con muy grand dolor" (st. 4). The soul admonishes the corpse for its sins in life:

> Desia contra el cuerpo: hereje, traydor,
> Del mal que fesiste, si eres repiso,
> Por tu bana-gloria e falso riso,
> Yo en el infierno biuo con dolor. (st. 3)

The Ánima specifically blames the Cuerpo it for its acts of greed, pride and lust in life. Furthermore, it goes on to acknowledge its own wish that it could also escape its eternal suffering in the Afterlife through finite death. "Mas me baldria contigo morir," wishes the soul, "Que non perseguir aquesto que sigo" (st. 6). Suddenly, in response, the inanimate corpse comes supernaturally to life to defend itself. Above all, there is a nihilistic sense of desperation in the words the revived corpse utters:

> (…) ¿por qué tanto culpar
> Me queres agora syn meresçimiento?
> Que sy dixe o fise por tu talento,
> Sy non mira agora qual es mi poder,
> Que estos gusanos non puedo toller,
> Que comen las carnes de mi criamiento. (st. 7)

After a second sequence of attack and counterattack by each speaker, the stalemate is ended with the appearance of a black demon that comes to claim the soul of the dead sinner.

> Ellos estando en esta porfia
> Salió vn diablo negro de vn espesura,
> Gesto espantable, de mala figura,
> Tynasas de fierro en las manos traya.
> Dixo contra el ánima: tu serás mia,
> E conmigo yrás allá a mi posada,
> Adonde serás bien aduergada,
> Que allá fallarás asás conpannia. (st. 12)

However, despite the demon's resolution to condemn the soul and carry it off to Hell, his attempt is thwarted by an Angel of God who wards him off claiming that "aquesta ánima será toda mia" (st. 13).[27] Before departing with the angel, the soul decries the vanities of the world making specific mention of numerous types of sins and the various social classes and professions that are subject to them. The work then ends with the Biblical adage: "eres çenisa, e çenisa te has de tornar" (st. 25).

Taken as a whole, the *Revelación de un hermitanno* reiterates many of the messages we have already learned to identify with works produced near the periods of plague epidemics. First, throughout the poem there is great emphasis placed upon the realistic characteristics of physical death and decay and this description includes the senses of both sight and smell. The *Cuerpo*, for example, is described as "holi[endo] muy mal" (st. 2) and was "leno de fedor e de grand calabrina" (st. 9). Unable to defend itself against the flies and worms that devour its flesh, the Cuerpo shows the effects of decay in places that are certainly the first to show signs of physical death. Thus, the corpse is described as having "ojos quebrados," "fas denegrida" and "barba cayda" (st. 2). Likewise, the Cuerpo suffers the attack of "gusanos e moscas" that "comen las carnes" at will. Such true-to-life portrayals of the physical effects of death have obvious plague associations; with the increase in contact with the dead and dying, Man would have developed a greater understanding of processes which accompany physical death. Although such realistic descriptions of human decay had appeared in pre-plague works of literature and art, scholars like Platt find that it is in the post-plague years that this subject is most plentiful and, subsequently, most effective and shocking. He concludes that death was "treated so realistically in many cases that they must at least imply more than usual familiarity with death's corruption" (151). In his opinion, the increased emphasis on the description of the cadaver, then, was directly related to widespread death caused by pestilence. However, despite obvious connections between plague and the increase in literary interest in physical decomposition, it is the second characteristic of plague literature—namely, its insistence on what Girard described as the "destruction of specificities"—that holds even greater interest for us.

Girard as well as Fass Leavy held as a principal distinguishing feature of plague literature the idea that such works characteristically show a tendency to destroy all forms of human distinctiveness. All social hierarchies are first transgressed and later completely abolished. A central theme to what we see in the *Dança general de la Muerte*, plague literature from Thucydides onward commonly portrays death as being able to overcome all obstacles and carry off any individual regardless of their social class or age. The *Revelación de un hermitanno* is no exception.

In what we consider to be a substantial amount of space dedicated to this theme in a short work, one can observe the impulse to enumerate fixed ranks of society that will be most conspicuously laid low by death.

> Veo que rreyes e enperadores,
> Papas, maestres e cardenales,
> Sus magnifiçençicas e pontificales,
> todos feneçen en banos sabores.
> Condes, duques, obispos, priores,
> Segund obraren, ansy gosarán,
> E los letrados entonçe verán
> Los malos juysios tornar en sabores. (st. 20)

As Florence Whyte has commented, the preceding lines are almost an exact summary of what we will later see in the *Dança general de la Muerte*.[28] This similarity is not surprising as Whyte concludes that "the two poems were written in the same general period and locality" (16). Such orderly naming of specific social classes that will be laid low by death, then, could have easily have mirrored the egalitarian message that was the harsh social byproduct of plague. The fact that the majority of the offices named pertain to members of the clergy can even be seen as a reference to the higher death rate and abandonment of parishes by the priesthood during pestilent times. Regardless of the criterion that led the anonymous poet to the inclusion or exclusion of the social classes he specifically mentions or does not mention, the lack of differentiation is clearly present. Taken in conjunction with what will be the final characteristic of plague literature—namely, the predilection for using macabre imagery based on the image of the putrefying corpse—one finds that it dovetails with the conception of death and dying that took on a new and more pessimistic meaning during this time period.

Throughout the *Revelación de un hermitanno*, there is an unmistakable emphasis on the macabre as one central means to underscore a didactic message that seeks to alert its intended audience to the need to tend the soul, which does not decay. From its opening setting in a "valle fondo, escuro, apartado, espesso de xaras," to its final admonition, "eres çeniza e en çeniza te has de tornar," the implied reader finds a greater desire to confront its philosophical and theological preoccupations, made grim and forceful through the use of much dark and macabre imagery. In a comparison of this poem with its alleged sources, Andrew M. Beresford finds that it is precisely the macabre innovations of the Castilian poem that sets it apart from any of its literary antecedents.

> The dark valley, a geographical concretization of the narrator's inner feelings, plays no part [in any previous source]; neither does the portrait of the rotting corpse, the winged soul metaphor, or even the use [sic] imagery associated with confinement and entrapment. (6)

The poet takes great pains to explicitly comment on the inability of the Body to defend itself from the "monton de gusanos" that devour its flesh (st. 22). Death is referred to as a cruel torturer that makes prisoners of its victims without mercy. The Ánima complains of a "muerte cruel" in which she suffers "atada en [una] prision" (st. 23; 10). The Devil, in what can be viewed as an extension of this torturer imagery, is described as having a "gesto espantable, de mala figura" and one who brings "tynasas de fierro en las manos" in order to confine its victims in Hell for all eternity (st. 12). Compared with the dominance of more optimistic religious works of the previous century—such as the *exemplum*-collections and the many Marian works written in the age of Alfonso X—these new images reflect a profound change in Man's relationship to death and dying. No longer the traditional idea of death—as the graceful elegiac sigh of the twelfth and thirteenth centuries—this new perception of death was now menacing and hideous. The perfect symbol for this new pessimistic vision, the putrefying corpse came to represent all the worst aspects of human mortality. There is an irrevocable connection between the body, which is time bound, and the soul, which is eternal and to focus on the physical deterioration of the body upon death is to deny the notion of eternal salvation.[29] Bodily disintegration and its visual predictability, therefore, are equated with the concept of nothingness after one's physical demise. A concept that implicitly denies the perpetual existence of the human soul, this thought would have stood in clear contrast with the tenets of traditional Christian dogma.

The idea of using the image of the animated corpse as a means of voicing the newly dominant, pessimistic view of death and dying comes as no surprise. For centuries, ascetic meditation had dwelt on dust and worms in an attempt to decry the frivolous pursuit of earthly pleasures in this life; numerous examples can be found in fifth century BC Greek grave epigrams and funeral paintings.[30] However, it is the unanticipated nature of death caused by plague that affords this sort of imagery its impact on popular literature. In Huizinga's view, this new literary motif had little to do with the fundamentals of Christian dogma.

> A thought which so strongly attaches to the earthly side of death can hardly be called truly pious. It would rather seem a kind of spasmodic reaction against an excessive sensuality. In exhibiting the horrors awaiting all human beauty, already lurking below the surface of corporeal charms, these preachers of contempt for the world express, indeed, a very materialistic sentiment, namely, that all beauty and all happiness are worthless *because* they are bound to end soon. Renunciation founded on disgust does not spring from Christian wisdom. (141)

The desire to invent an image that embodied the darker side of human mortality led to the ideas with strong graphic modes of representation. There is no tenderness in the image of the decomposing corpse, and the consoling idea of "death as the final rest and end of all suffering" is absent altogether in the *Revelación*. At its roots, the macabre vision is entirely self-seeking. "It is hardly the absence of the departed dear ones that is deplored," comments Huizinga, "it is the fear of one's own death, and this only is seen as the worst of evils" (150). The terror of the sentient corpse unable to defend itself against the worms of the grave stands in direct conflict with and contrast to the concept of the resurrection of Christ who promises salvation of the faithful from eternal death. It is precisely for this reason that Binski characterizes late medieval culture as one that was "inseparable from individualism," for the rise of the macabre image also brought with it an "awareness and desperate love of this life" (131). Although such views certainly existed in the period preceding the Iberian plagues of the mid fourteenth-century, it is only in the shadow of mortal epidemic disease that this concern with decay develops to reach its artistic and expressive summit.

La dança general de la Muerte

From the earliest studies of European literature produced after the Black Death, scholars have insisted that the most direct example of how widespread plague epidemics influenced the literature and art of the time is found in the various manifestations of the theme of the Dance of Death. Raymond Crawfurd's 1914 study, *Plague and Pestilence in Literature and Art,* is one such example of this critical opinion that is still prevalent today. After studying pure literature, art and what he terms "medical literature"—a term he applies to the type of medical treatises presented earlier in this study—Crawfurd concludes that plague's influence on literature and art is unquestionable and that its psychological effects can be found in numerous literary and artistic forms.

> For three centuries and more after the Black Death plague was endemic throughout central and southern Europe, and its presence is indelibly recorded in the productions of contemporary art. Dances of Death, plague banners, votive and commemorative paintings, and actual representations of plague scenes all bear silent testimony to the abiding presence of the enemy within the gates. *Memento mori*, with its dismal foreboding, was the appropriate motto of the age. Innocent III in his *De Contemptu Mundi* had said the last word on the misery of human existence, and the shame and degradation of the human body, polluted and polluting, long before the Black Death: but henceforward the gloom that haunted the soul of this great successor of St. Peter seems to diffuse itself throughout the world. (133)

The theme of the Dance of Death, then, can be seen as one distinct version of a larger group of literary imaginings that all reflect morbid medieval attitudes with regard to death and the grave. As such, if one is to understand the true meaning behind the theme of the Dance of Death, it is necessary to detail its evolution with respect to macabre literature in general. And, as we shall see, the theme of the Dance of Death—similar to what we have seen in the medical treatises produced around the periods of widespread plague infection—also suffered a gradual transformation that moved from a general portrayal of an image to the distinct and wholly individualistic personification of Death itself. As it is specifically the *image* of Death found in works such as the *Dança general*—not necessarily any strong historical or literary narrative—that presently calls our attention, we will first observe how this stylized image functioned previous to the Black Death in order to better understand the changes of the post-plague years.

As previously noted, it is a particular human characteristic to employ the use of an image as a means to represent that which is profoundly incomprehensible. Indeed, death is one such event and, as such, it is not surprising that Man has attempted to visualize it through art and literature since antiquity. Karl S. Guthke, in *The Gender of Death*, asserts that it is this sort of image making that actually *defines* humans for the creative process is a necessary impulse with a clear psychological purpose.

> The fact that some religions try to curb [image-making] only shows that it is basic to our orientation in the world. This urge to make an image is activated most dramatically whenever we experience situations that baffle or overwhelm us because familiar patterns of thought cannot cope with them, cannot give them shape and order that make them familiar. Death is such an experience—our own death and that of others (...) Imagination, being the elementary urge to visualize, does not stop short of the "unimaginable." It gives shape to the shapeless by approximating it to the familiar, thereby endowing it with meaning. At the border of intelligibility, the imagination (...) transforms the unintelligible into an image that clarifies, elucidates, and thereby renders accessible to understanding what seemed to elude it. (8–9)

Death, the ultimate human mystery, is made concrete through use of the image and—just as our imagination is limitless—so are the many representations of this biological phenomenon. Death personified as the Grim Reaper with scythe in hand, as the classical Thanatos of Greek mythology (known as Orcus to the Romans) and as the Book of Revelations "rider on a pale horse" all come readily to mind.[31] In fact, for nearly every culture that has ever existed, there is some sort of personification or anthropomorphism of death and that image is typically one that is based on human—not animal—form. Guthke has also demonstrated that this visualization of Death in human form shows no correlation with the grammatical gender of the word 'death' and is more likely to have followed literary and historical antecedents. Thus, 'la muerte' in Spanish literary works such as those by Cervantes and Calderón are easily portrayed as male figures while in the Germanic languages of Scandinavia, the word was grammatically masculine up until the Middle Ages despite the numerous feminine literary and artistic representations of the image of Death (24–29). Irrespective of the grammatical gender of the word 'death,' the most important factor for the literary writer was the ability to make an instant connection with his intended audience. Thus, in trying to render comprehensible the profound mystery of death for didactic or other purposes, giving Death a human form was a logical occurrence. However, while literary antecedents to the Spanish *Dança general de la Muerte* may have indeed employed a similar use of visualizing Death in human form, it is not until the post Black Death years that we see such sophistication of the image. Where early medieval representations of Death commonly emphasized its powerlessness—such as the Worms missal of the eleventh century where Death cowers on its back beneath Christ the victor[32]—, post-Black Death personifications are decidedly more sophisticated and terrifying. Often portrayed in skeletal form, Death in the fifteenth century typically connects with his audience by adopting the high fashion and habits of individual members of society.[33] With its altogether pessimistic tone and consistent highlighting of the individual rather than society, the Spanish *Dança general de la Muerte* is also a good reflection of this changing sentiment regarding death and dying.

The Spanish *Dança general de la Muerte* is based on a literary motif with a long cultural history, so if we are to understand how this specific work represents the changing opinions on human mortality in Spain when it was written, we must also take into account how scholarly opinion has considered this work within the larger European context. With this purpose in mind, Alan Deyermond's *A Literary History of Spain: the Middle Ages*, provides a concise overview of the entire Dance of Death genre:

> An increasing concern with death and its physical consequences is a feature of the late Middle Ages, and its most characteristic manifestation is the Dances of Death. In most countries, these poems accompany a series of pictures (paintings in churches or on the walls of cemeteries, woodcuts in block-books) which show skeletons seizing representatives of the different ranks of society and dragging them into the dance; worms and decomposing corpses are a frequent feature of the illustrations (...). The European Dances of Death seem to have begun in the fourteenth century, and are connected with the general pessimism of the late Middle Ages, which had a variety of causes, including the economic and demographic collapse caused by the Black Death. The sermons in which the travelling friars sought to urge men to repentance involved a concentration on death, and especially on its negative aspects. No satisfactory literary source has been found for the Dances of Death, whose real origin is in the social and intellectual background. (190–91)[34]

Although scholars have yet to identify conclusive literary antecedents to the Dances of Death, there are a number of interesting and convincing theories as to the origin and development of this well-known motif. In 1892, Wilhelm Seelmann published *Die Totentänze des Mittelalters*—an essay that sought to provide a listing of all known literature and artwork that depicted the Dance of Death. After careful analysis, his conclusion was that all the diverse works that he collected stemmed from one original French source or "urtext"—an archetype that has never been found.[35]

To date, many critics have taken a stance either supporting or refuting Seelmann's theory. Commenting strictly on the Spanish *Dança general de la Muerte*, Robert Felkel's 1973 Ph.D. dissertation summarizes the trajectory of scholarly opinion as to the genesis of the Spanish version in relation to the theories offered by Seelman:

> Seelman (...) maintained that a French morality play was the starting-point of the Spanish *Dança general*, as well as the Paris *Danse macabre* and the Lübeck *Totentanz*. (...) Karl Künstle, on the other hand, (...) prefers to see the origin of the Dance of Death in the Legend of the Three Living and the Three Dead. He therefore follows the ideas of P. Vigo,[36] who was the first to print a twelfth century poem on this subject preserved in a manuscript of Ferrara. A similar emphasis on folkloric elements distinguishes the theory developed by W. Fehse in his book *Der Ursprung der Totentänze*.[37] He noticed a discrepancy between the texts and the paintings of the Dance of Death: in the former a single figure of Death speaks, whereas in the latter there are many skeletons represented. (...) O. Ursprung's article[38] anticipates future research by postulating a Catalonian origin for the Dances of Death. (...) His theories would be partially confirmed later by Florence Whyte and (...) by José María Solá-Solé. (...) Miss Whyte refutes Seelman's theory that the *Dança general* is a translation of a lost French original and argues instead that traces of a peninsular background are abundant. (1–3)[39]

Modern criticism, while not fully embracing the assertion that the Spanish *Dança general* evolved in a manner wholly independent of direct European influence, tends to follow Whyte's lead in trying to identify possible peninsular influences on this motif. For example, J.T. Snow takes the three basic elements of the *Dança general* as detailed by Whyte— namely, (1) the dance, (2) the procession of victims that follow an arrangement by estate, and (3) the inevitability of physical death—and makes a convincing argument that ties it to Alfonso X's Cantiga 409. Furthermore, in his recent comprehensive study of the evolution of the Medieval Danzas de la Muerte, Víctor Infantes highlights this same question of literary antecedents to the Spanish *Dança general* in exhaustive work in his preliminary explanation as to his particular selection of texts:

> (...) debería disculparme de antemano por la pretensión de mostrar unas obras que no siempre tendrán una relación expresa con las Danzas de la Muerte y, al decir expresa, me refiero a una relación *evidente* y *mensurable*; igualmente, tampoco ofrecen en muchos casos una relación integral entre ellos mismos. Su vigencia y difusión es más que discutible en muchas ocasiones y los caminos recorridos para su conocimiento, sinuosos y laberínticos; de ahí que no podamos establecer rigurosamente—por lo menos hasta donde llegan nuestros conocimientos y capacidades—vías de interrelación mutua (y de su confluencia con las Danzas de la Muerte) con suficiente seguridad. No todos derivan de un *modelo literario* común, que a mi modo de ver no existe, sino de una *sensibilidad compartida* hacia el tema macabro, que los aúna desde esta perspectiva crítica, pero que tal vez quede muy lejos de la *realidad literaria* de su momento. (59–60)

Similar to what we saw earlier in this chapter in the theories of Girard, who argues that all plague literature inherently contains shared sensitivities with regard to the treatment of Death and the individual, Infantes develops his argument and uses it to select specific texts in order to demonstrate peninsular antecedents to the *Dança general*. This theory, also based on the idea of "shared sensitivities," is used by Infantes in a manner that can accommodate the inclusion of both direct and *indirect* sources to the Spanish analogs.

Despite the inability to conclusively determine specific precursors of the *Dança general*, it is certainly the case that the Spanish version of the Dance of Death is not the first creative work to deal with the topic of human mortality. Léonard P. Kurtz, along with critics such as Künstle, Whyte and Tristram, believe that the Spanish *Dança general* derived from previous well known representations such as carved or painted figures on coffins and popular tales such as the "Legend of the Three Living and the Three Dead." Kurtz offers evidence of Roman wine jars and drinking cups dating from the first century A.D. that portray jubilant skeletons engaging in the same acts of dancing and merriment that one would expect during a celebration. However, in this scholar's opinion, it is the tone of these early artifacts—compared to those closer to the time of the European Black Death—that sparks the greatest interest.

> Death was never cloaked with more modesty than during the XIIIth century. Nothing more soothing or pleasant can be imagined than certain figures engraved on funeral slabs or tombs. Hands joined, eyes open, these beautiful young dead seem to participate already in eternal life. Far from causing death to be feared, they almost caused it to be liked. (7)

This mode of representing Death is clearly in contrast with the harsh, realistic and eminently pessimistic representations of Death that we see in works such as the *Dança general*. As a means of comparison, Huizinga's description of tomb sculptures in the post Black Death years clearly illustrates the drearier new ideologies concerning death and dying:

> Ascetic meditation had, in all ages, dwelt on dust and worms. The treatises on the contempt of the world had, long since, evoked all the horrors of decomposition, but it is only towards the end of the fourteenth century that pictorial art, in its turn, seizes upon this motif. To render the horrible details of decomposition, a realistic force of expression was required, to which painting and sculpture only attained towards 1400. At the same time, the motif spread from ecclesiastical to popular literature. Until far into the sixteenth century, tombs are adorned with hideous images of a naked corpse with clenched hands and rigid feet, gaping mouth and bowels crawling with worms. The imagination of those times relished these horrors, without ever looking one stage further, to see how corruption perishes in its turn, and flowers grow where it lay.(140–41)

Likewise, the *Dança general* shows a similar emphasis on the harsher aspects of Death. From the very beginning of the work, Death is described as a demanding master who, when shooting its life-robbing "frecha cruel," proudly declares "pues non ay tan fuerte nin rezio gigante / que deste mi arco se puede anparar" (st. 1).[40] Explicit in its reference to plague, Death attacks with "corrupçión de landre o carbonico"—a fate from which neither young nor old "por cosa ninguna que sea escapar" (st. 2 / 7).[41] Despite the efforts of beautiful maidens who try to elude Death through use of "flores e rosas"—another common practice in the prevention of pestilential disease—unwavering Death steals them away to make them his brides (st 9). Instead of fine clothes as wedding gifts, he promises "sepulcros escuros de dentro fedientes / e por los manjares, gusanos royentes / que coman de dentro su carne podrida" (St. 10). In comparison with earlier representations such as Roman artifacts and early tomb decorations, examples such as these make it clear that the Spanish Dance of Death stands out for its general lack of compassion or tenderness. These new sensibilities concerning death are equally apparent when comparing a work such as the *Dança genral* to the Legend of the Three Living and the Three Dead.

Tristram is among one of many scholars who has argued that the admonitory Legend of the Three Living and the Three Dead could possibly be a direct antecedent to the motif of the Dance of the Dead. The Legend, found in diverse forms throughout most Western European cultures, can be can be summarized as follows:

> (...) it is essentially the encounter between three living men and three animate skeletons who address the Living with the words: 'What you are, so once were we; what we are, so shall you be.' The core of the Legend never varies, though time adds to it certain embellishments: the Living may, for example, be gaily dressed youths, or kings, or be distinguished into the three Ages; they are often engaged in hunting, occasionally with hounds, but more often with falcons, for falconry was, *par excellence*, the sport of the nobility. The Dead are less easily differentiated (...). (Tristram, 162)

Despite the similar use of imagery in giving Death a human form, what is noteworthy here is the lack of differentiation among the animate skeletons that come to give their warnings to the Living. Clearly, in the Legend, the use of the animate Dead serve another purpose when compared with the *Dança general*. They do not necessarily need to be distinguished by age or estate as they function on a more didactic or moral level admonishing the Living—and, as a consequence the intended audience—to conduct themselves in this life in a manner befittingthe faithful who wish to gain entrance into Paradise. This underlying message of *choice*, prompting Man to reform in this life or suffer the consequences in the next, is something altogether absent in the *Dança general*.

The figure of Death in the *Dança general de la Muerte* is remarkable both for the depth of imagination in which this—the idea of the physiological mystery surrounding human mortality—is conveyed as well as for the underlying and more pessimistic ideological message Death has for its audience. In comparison with other death-related themes such as the Legend of the Three Living and the Three Dead, it is clear that the anonymous author of the *Dança general* makes a distinct conceptual break from works that represent Death as an animate corpse.

With grim determination, Death is presented again and again as an unstoppable force that pays no heed to either the social class or desperate pleas of its victims. The Padre Santo laments:

> ¡Ay de mí triste, qué cosa tan fuerte
> a [mí] que tractava tan grand perlazía!
> ¡aver de pasar agora la muerte
> e non me valer lo que dar solía!
>
> Benefiçios e honrras e grand sennoría
> tove en el mundo pensando vevir;
> pues de ti, muerte, non puedo fuir,
> ¡Valme Jhesu Cristo, e tú, Virgen María! (St. 12)

Far from the early medieval image we previously saw of a powerless being that cowers under the will of Christ, Death is now portrayed as a fear-inspiring unstoppable force. For example, the Enperador complains that he is taken "a fuerça" to Death's dance and that "non ay ningund rey nin duque esforçado que della me pueda agora defender" (St 14). Later, Death slays both King and Duke despite attempts to defend themselves by force or by pleas for mercy. The King declares "non querría ir a tan baxa dança" and therefore desperately calls for his cavalleros to defend him "por fuerça de lança" (st. 18). Likewise, the Duke unsuccessfully begs "¡espérame un poco, muerte, yo te ruego! / Si non te detienes, miedo he que luego / me prendas o me mates" (st 22). Thus, where we see the pre-Black Death animate skeleton functioning as a warning to spur mankind into acts of reformation in this life, Death as portrayed in the *Dança general* violently rips life from her victims regardless of whatever pleas or concessions they might offer.[42]

Scholars have also noted that it is both the physical appearance as well as the conduct of Death in the *Dança general* that combine to support the new harsher image of death as an unstoppable and fearful process. Physically, the seventy-nine stanzas and short prose prologue describe Death in traditionally horrific terms:

> Sex is implied in line 72: mas non puede ser, que son mis esposas, and in line 259: abraçad mi: agora seredes mi esposo. Death has teeth: como la muerte con sus duros dientes (line 159) and harsh hands: la muerte con su mano dura, (line 221), and her face is ugly: ca el thannedor trahe feo visaje, (line 204). (White, 51)

When compared with the beautiful dances of the "lindas donzellas, / de duennas fermosas de alto linaje," the Condestable immediately recognizes that Death's frightful appearance indicates that her "dance" will be decidedly different. Psychologically as well, Death's ugly intentions are made clear through the use of dialogue; Death is clearly the central figure and, consequently, the entity that enjoys absolute control of movement throughout the work. In other words, "es ella la que domina y subyuga a los mortales, no tanto como instrumento de Dios y su justicia, sino como meta final y punto de llegada (Solá-Solé, *Dança*, 16). Death still contains an adumbrative message regarding Man's specific end; however, rather than inciting men to choose between the religiously sanctioned ideas of right and wrong, the personification of Death in the *Dança general* forces humans to submit without mercy and without specific reference to an Afterlife. The fact that Death moves systematically through the social Estates of Man without regard for age – she openly declares that neither a "ninno de días" nor a "viejo inpotente" can stop her progress—or gender—her first victims are female while the majority are male—only serves to reinforce this point (st. 3 / 9). Thus, much in the same way that the social effects of plague led to a greater concern for self-preservation at the expense of the community, so also does the terrifying representation of Death in the *Dança general* emphasize the individual impotence of each victim in his efforts to avert his fate.

Notes

1. See Millard Meiss, *Painting in Florence and Sienna After the Black Death* (Princeton: Princeton UP, 1978).
2. Found in the supplementary material included in the appendix to Daniel Defoe, *A Journal of the Plague Year*, edited by Paula R. Backscheider (New York: W. W. Norton and Company, 1992): 197–198.
3. Gyug clarifies: "These numbers include only resignations that do not specify a new appointee. Documents dealing with the provision to benefices vacant through resignation also increase from 3.3 per month to 4.3 per month."
4. Gyug, "The Effects and Extent of the Black Death," p. 395.
5. See René Girard, "The Plague in Literature and Myth," *Theories of Myth: From Ancient Israel and Greece to Freud, Jung, Campbell and Levi-Strauss*, (New York: Garland, 1996): 162.
6. The persecution of the Jewish people in Spain around the time of the Black Death is supported by extensive documentation and, according to Gottfried, the years 1348 to 1350 saw the Jews of Castile and Aragon reduced to one-quarter its former size. See Sobrequés Callicó pp. 80–81; Horrox pp. 222–223; and Gottfried pp. 52–53 for further information.
7. See René Girard, *The Scapegoat* (Baltimore: Johns Hopkins UP, 1986): 2–3.
8. It must also be noted that literary references to disease in general often spur great controversy among critics today. As contemporary authors, such as the anonymous author of the *Dança general de la Muerte*, lacked medical training, their accounts are often imprecise with their vocabulary and lacking in precise descriptions of the infirmity. Josiah C. Russell, one scholar who has spent considerable time trying to distinguish one disease from another by way of textual analysis, concludes that it is often impossible to determine which terms refer to plague as terms for it often applied to two other common epidemic diseases: smallpox and dysentery (See "That Earlier Plague"). Likewise, many other scholars confuse the matter even further by disregarding altogether that such a possibility for ambiguity even exists. In 1997, for example, María Inés Chamorro Fernández published a work by Joan de Angulo titled "De las bubas…". Her first two pages attempt a brief summary of the use of the term "buba:"

> las *bubas* o búas, (…) parecen derivar de un regresivo *bubón* "tumor voluminoso" en particular el de peste. Esta palabra está documentada

> en la *Danza de la Muerte* (1400) y se aplica a sífilis junto con el término *landre* "bellota", "buba". En el *Glosario de Palacio* significa "infarto inguinal". En el *Corbacho* se dice "peste levantina". Nebrija escribe <<landre que mata con pestilencia: glándula>> y <<landres del cuello>> con el significado de "peste con bubas". (7)

> While she is certainly right to name syphilis as the culprit in some of her examples, it would be premature to prove that this affliction was behind all the texts in question without additional research.

9. From a reprint found in A Journal of the Plague Year, Edited by Paula R. Backscheider (New York: W. W. Norton and Company, 1992): 211–212.
10. In the Decameron, Boccaccio describes grisly scenes that would have surely been similar to what occurred in Spain given the comparable conditions:

    > Whenever people died, their neighbours nearly always followed a single, set routine, prompted as much by their fear of being contaminated by the decaying corpse as by any charitable feelings they may have entertained towards the deceased. Either on their own, or with the assistance of bearers whenever those were to be had, they extracted the bodies of the dead from their houses and left them lying outside their front doors, where anyone going about the streets, especially in the early morning, could have observed countless numbers of them (56).

11. The sources from which Gyug supports his conclusions are detailed in note 7 of "Effects and Extent," 392. Curiously, he also theorizes that the manner in which the documents were written are also indicative of the frantic conditions of the time. While in pre-plague years he finds that the script of such registers were "carefully spaced and written copies," post-plague entries suffer in terms of its legibility and its spacing (394). The argument follows that if the scribes demonstrated the effects of the desperate conditions in which they worked, one can only imagine the state of the rest of the religious community.
12. Symbolic associations between inanimate objects and the Holy family were frequent in the pictorial representations of early Byzantine Art such as in the apse mosaic from Sant' Apollinare in Classe (See Gardner's *Art Throught the Ages—Tenth Edition*, Fort Worth: Harcourt Brace, 1996): 299. For further information on how the architectural design of religious places of try to imitate Paradise, see the discussion of Mircea Elaide, *The Sacred & the Profane: The Nature of Religion*, (San Diego: Harcourt Brace, 1987): 60–61.
13. This is the date established in Ramón Menéndez Pidal's *Romancero hispánico, 1* (Madrid: Espasa-Calpe, 1953): 102; later reaffirmed in José María Viña Liste's *Cronología de la literatura española*, 63. It must also be noted that Jane E. Connolly,

in her edition of the *Libro de miseria*, advocates an earlier date of composition for the poem. In her estimation, the work is "the product not of the late fourteenth century, as most critics contend, but of the last years of the thirteenth century or the first years of the fourteenth" (223). In support of this dating, she offers various examples of a lexical and social nature that she believes establishes her claim. However, subsequent reactions to Connolly have refuted her theory and, instead, advocate the traditional dating of the late fourteenth century as established by the vast majority of scholars. One such example is the opinion of Nicasio Salvador Miguel who, in a scathing review of her book (*Hispanic Review*, 56 (1988), 495–496), concludes that "pese al singular interés con que uno sigue estas indagaciones [las de Connolly], se queda muy lejos del asentimiento." Miguel goes on to cite examples of how Connolly bases her conclusions on "atestaciones sobre métrica necesitadas de absoluta revisión" and her blatant adulteration and/or unfamiliarity with previously published work on the subject (496).

14. This anonymous poem is also known as: *Proverbios en rimo del sabio Salomón, rey de Israel* and *Proverbios de Salomón*. For more information, see Alan Deyermond, *A Literary History of Spain: the Middle Ages* (London: Ernest Benn, 1971): 108–109; "Proverbios de Salamón", *Homenaje a Menéndez Pidal*, I, Ed. C.E. Kany (Madrid: Hernando, 1925): 269–285.

15. Despite basing many works upon original Latin sources, Brian Dutton has affirmed the creative merits of Berceo in various critical studies. Among such studies are included: *La vida de Santo Domingo de Silos* (London: Tamesis, 1978), 181–254; *El sacrificio de la misa. La vida de Santa Oria. El martirio de San Lorenzo* (London: Tamesis, 1981), 76–80 and 164–80; *El duelo de la Virgen. Los himnos. Los loores de nuestra Señora. Los signos del Juicio Final* (London: Tamesis, 1975), 135–44; *La vida de San Mill'an de Congolla* (London: Tamesis, 1967), 197–235; *Los milagros de nuestra Senora* (London: Tamesis, 1971).

16. Ricardo Ciérvide, "Notas en torno al *Libro de miseria de omne:* lo demoniaco e infernal en el códice," *Estudios de Deusto*, 22 (1974): 81. Francisco López Estrada, *Introducción a la literatura medieval española*, 4th ed, (Madrid: Gredos, 197): 375. Dámaso Alonso, *De los siglos oscuros al de oro: notas y artículos a través de 700 años de letras españolas*, (Madrid: Gredos, 1958): 110. Rosa Bobes Naves, *Clerecía y juglaria en el siglo XIV: "Libro de buen amor,"* (Madrid: Cincel, 1980): 74.

17. See, for example: Robert E. Lewis, ed., *De Miseria Condicionis Humane* (Athens, Georgia: U Georgia P, 1978): 3–30; Donald R. Howard, ed., *On the Misery of the Human Condition: De Miseria Humane Conditionis* (Indianapolis: Bobbs-Merrill Co., 1969): xiii–xx.

18. Achille Luchaire, *Innocent III: Rome et l'Italie* (Paris: Librairie Hachette et Cie., 1907): 10.

19. Antonio Viscardi, *Saggio sulla letteratura religiosa del medio evo romanzo* (Padova: Pubblicazione della Facultà di Lettere e Filosofia della R. Università di Padova, 1932): 67.
20. All quotations from the *Libro de miseria d'omne* are from the Connolly edition. Citations are made using standard verse references.
21. See Hans Robert Jauss, *Toward an Aesthetic of Reception*, Trans. Timothy Bahti. Theory and History of Literature, 2 (Minneapolis: U of Minnesota P, 1982): 101–102.
22. For more information on this work, see Alan Deyermond, *A Literary History*, 72–76; and *Medieval Debate Poetry*, Ed. and Tran. Michel-André Bossy, (New York: Garland, 1987).
23. In his recent article, Andrew M. Beresford readdresses the issue of the sources of the *Revelación de un hermitanno* and its sister work, the *Disputa del cuerpo e del ánima*. While he claims that the innovations of each work allow for it to be considered an independent product of creative art, there is also a great likelihood that the *Visión de Filiberto* was the primary source of the later poems (11).
24. This dating of this work is taken from the internal reference as well as the earliest known publication as established by José María Viña Liste, *Cronología de la literatura espanola, I) Edad media*, (Madrid: Cátedra, 1991): 67.
25. For more on debate poetry, see Raby: 283–340.
26. All citations of this work are from the Biblioteca Escorial codex as reproduced in *Poetas anteriores al siglo XV*: 387–388. I cite by verse number.
27. It must be noted that a second version of this poem, called the *Disputa del cuerpo e del anima*, ends with an even gloomier resolution. Although sharing in the *Revalación*'s beginning, introductory dream, description of the rotting corpse and vigorous debate between the body and the soul, the *Disputa del cuerpo e del anima* concludes with the soul being carried off by the devil. As both poems shared a common date of composition and were similar in content and style, it would have also been possible to select this second manuscript as a primary source of plague literature. However, as Deyermond points out, the version called the *Revelación* "shares some features with the *Danza de la Muerte* (*Middle Ages*, 189). As such, it seemed the more logical choice for this study.
28. See The Dance of Death in Spain and Catalonia (New York: Arno, 1977): 15.
29. This notion is developed further by Barbara I. Gusick, 315–330.
30. See Emily Vermeule, 42–82.
31. For more information on the various representations of death, see Guthke's first chapter: "Imagining the Unimaginable: Death Personified," pp. 7–37.
32. See Guthke, 45.
33. This new graphic representation of Death is especially noticeable in the illuminated manuscripts of the era. For more information, see Sandra L.

Hindman's discussion in *The Danse Macabre of Women*, Ed. Ann Tukey Harrison, (Kent: Kent State UP, 1994): 15–43.

34. For purposes of clarification and expansion of this description, it is also useful to acknowledge the recent definition of the Dances as offered by Víctor Infantes for—as he rightly asserts—far too many critics simply ignore any formal definition of the motif as commonplace. In Infantes' definition, the Dances of Death are defined as: "una sucesión de texto e imágenes presididas por la Muerte como personaje central—generalmente representada por un esqueleto, un cadáver o un vivo en descomposición—y que, en actitud de danzar, dialoga y arrastra uno por uno a una relación de personajes habitualmente representativos de las diferentes clases sociales" (21).

35. For more discussion on Seelman, see White, ix; Felkel, 1; and Clark, 336.

36. P. Vigo, *Le Danze Macabre in Italia*, 2nd ed. (Bergamo, 1901). Discussed by White, *Dance of Death*, 46.

37. W. Fehse, *Der Ursprung der Totentänze* (Halle, 1907). Discussed by Whyte, *Dance of Death*, 46.

38. O. Ursprung, "Spanisch-katalanische Liedkunst des 14. Jahrhundert," *Zeitschrift fur Musikwissenschaft* 4 (1921–22): 136–160. Discussed by José María Solá-Solé in his "En torno a la *Dança general de la Muerte*," *Hispanic Review* 36 (1968): 313.

39. Of the more interesting theories against a peninsular source to the *Dança general* is that if Menéndez y Pelayo who claims that the gloom inherent to the Dance was abated by the strong sunshine of Castile:

> La Danza de la Muerte es entre nosotros concepción totalmente exótica, y de la cual ningun [sic] rastro hallamos en Castilla hasta la presente obra [i.e. la *Dança general*], ni en Cataluña hasta que en época aun más tardía (…) No parece sino que la alegría y la luz de nuestro cielo; y el espíritu realista de la misma devoción peninsular ahuyentaban de España como de Italia estas visiones macabras (…) que en regiones mas nebulosas, en Alemania y en el norte de Francia, informan un ciclo entero de composiciones artísticas (…) ni arraigó ni podía arraigar en España. (from Whyte, x–xi)

40. All quotations from *La dança general de la Muerte* are from the siglo XV edition of Víctor Infantes. I cite by strophe.

41. The explicit references to plague in the *Dança general de la Muerte* is forcefully presented by Marcelino Amasuno in his article "La medicina y el físico en *La dança general de la Muerte*." For specific textual examples, see pages 10–13.

42. It is interesting to note that this pitiless and unwavering imposition of Death's will is exactly the same scenario that we previously described with regard to the

identification and subsequent condemnation of diseased individuals into pesthouses.

Conclusion

In 1938, Charles Verlinden published one of the most conservative assessments of the general impact of medieval plague in Spain as well as in Europe as a whole. Despite his acknowledged lack of any objective, quantifiable data concerning actual mortality rates or nominal economic loss, he concluded:

> The great plague caused considerable disturbance in Spain but no real changes in the fundamental character of any political, social, or economic institution. If it momentarily retarded economic evolution, it did not modify the orientation of this evolution. Moreover, we believe that this is a conclusion that is valid for all of Europe. (Bowsky, 143–146)

Currently, this opinion could not be more strongly opposed. Alongside a re-assessment and consequent discovery of new sources of information from which to extrapolate more accurate mortality figures (such as those mentioned in the Introduction), there has been a corresponding increase in critical attention paid to forms of information long-overlooked by scholars of plague. Among these rank the important studies of the Barcelona Diocese registries by Richard Gyug, the Aragonese legal documents published by Amanda López de Meneses and the recent medical treatises published by both Marcelino Amasuno and María Nieves Sánchez. Despite the fact that most historians still openly admit that compiling accurate mortality figures from medieval sources is "virtually impossible," even the most conservative Black Death figures based on these new sources of information now place the death rate at one third of the population within two years at the very *minimum*.[1] Undoubtedly, this figure is itself alarmingly high. Taking into account that it was the recurring plague epidemics—rather than the single 1347–1348 Black Death outbreak—that led to the widespread distress of a population whose numbers suffered constant downturns, this calamity most certainly would have had enormous influence on the society in which it occurred.[2] The debates over the last fifty years have just now begun to indicate how much of the answer to this perplexing question of plague impact can be found in the medical and literary productions of the time.[3]

When the historian Francis Aidan Gasquet published his 1893 study in which he affirmed that the pandemic killed off approximately one-half of the population where it occurred, the immediate consequence of such a high estimated death toll was the portrayal of medieval plague as an apocalyptic scourge which by itself triggered a series of fundamental cultural changes. For example, with such extremely high mortality rates in mind, Gasquet concluded that the two largest groups to be affected would have been the laborers and the clergy:

> The sudden sweeping away of the population and the consequent scarcity of labourers, raised, it is well recognised, new and extravagant expectations in the minds of the lower classes; or, to use a modern expression, labour began then to understand its value and assert its power. (...) in 1351 the whole ecclesiastical system was wholly disorganised, or indeed, more than half ruined, and that everything had to be built up anew. As regards education, the effect of the catastrophe on the body of the clergy was prejudicial beyond the power of calculation. To secure the most necessary public ministrations of the rites of religion the most inadequately-prepared subjects had to be accepted, and even these could be obtained only in insufficient numbers. The immediate effect on the people was a religious paralysis. Instead of turning men to God the scourge turned them to dispair, and this not only in England, but in all parts of Europe. (xxii)

Of course, with the extremely high mortality rates upon which Gasquet based his conclusions, it was much easier to imagine the cataclysmic changes that the pestilence would have caused. The rapid death of one-half of any population would certainly translate into sweeping and profound changes at all levels of society. However, as Gasquet's figures were subsequently refuted by scholars such as Levett, Russell and Shrewsbury, the perception of the plague's impact suffered in a similar fashion—lower death rates were simply translated into lower overall effects of the disease. Hence, the conclusions of researchers such as Verlinden who claimed that the pestilence caused "considerable disturbance" in Spain and the rest of Europe but had no fundamental effect of changing any major social institution (90).

Currently, scholars of plague have begun to calculate the effects of years of debate and no longer assume—as did their predecessors—that higher plague mortality figures are in direct correlation with the greater overall cultural impact of the disease. Although our modern perceptions of the death rate directly attributed to plague have drastically increased as a result of new sources of information, most critics now understand that the true effects of the pestilential infection can no longer be as easily identified as once believed. Horrox is one of many scholars who has begun to recognize that the social and psychological effects of plague do not necessarily translate directly into abrupt cultural changes.

> The original exponents of a one in two death rate took it for granted that the enormous mortality would mean enormous change; just as their critics assumed that modest change must be evidence of modest mortality. That simple correlation no longer exists. In the cultural arena it is now more widely recognized that people under pressure are likely to articulate their anxieties in ways which are already familiar to them, and that cultural continuities spanning the plague cannot therefore be taken as evidence for the insignificance of those anxieties, or of the upheaval which triggered them. Terror is not any less real because it fails to find novel ways of expressing itself—indeed, the reverse is more likely to be true. (236)

This having been noted, it is easy to understand why more scholars of plague studies are returning to medieval writings of both a medical and literary nature; they are a direct reflection of the calamitous time period that inspired their genesis. These writings are the best way to gain clearer insights as to how widespread plague could have influenced modes of thought. It is within these works, regardless of their lack or inclusion of the "cultural continuities" which preceded them, that one will discover the true effects of Medieval plague. With regard to Medieval Spain, this specific desire to further explore human reactions to the disease was also the underlying criterion which governed the selection of both the medical and literary texts considered in this study. It is only through the treatment of their similarities—while keeping in mind both their historical and literary contexts—that one can fully begin to understand the human reactions of their individual authors.

Despite obvious differences in subject matter and compositional purpose, Girard was one of the first scholars to recognize that all forms of writing produced near the times of pestilential outbreaks all share definite similarities. As he concludes, these similarities exist regardless of the specific nature of the writing in question or their country of origin.

> (...) there is a strange uniformity to the various treatments of the plague, not only literary and mythical but also scientific and non-scientific, of both past and present. Between the matter-of-fact, or even statistical account of Defoe in his Journal of the Plague Year and the near hysteria of Artaud in Le Théâtre et la peste, the differences, at close range, turn out to be minor. (155)

With this in mind, it is valid to consider—as we have done—works as chronologically distant such as those of Thucydides and Procopius along side later literary writings such as the *Dança general de la Muerte*. All were produced during the time of epidemic contamination and, as such, are inherently related to one another through the common link of this recurring biological disaster. In a very real sense, it is the reaction of these early authors to the plagues of antiquity that serves as the frame to which all later forms of plague writing currently conform. Paul Slack describes these universal similarities as follows:

> Almost all epidemics were seen by contemporaries, for example, as being transmitted from person to person and as arising from particular, usually filthy, local conditions: notions of 'contagion' and 'miasma', of a more or less undefined kind, were combined. Again and again 'stench' lay at the root of the disease. Common social responses—and intellectual justifications for them—followed from these assumptions. Flight from an infected place was usual, and had to be defended (or attacked) since it took people away from charitable, neighbourly or political duties. Carriers of disease were identified and scapegoats stigmatised: foreigners most often (...) If social prejudices became polarised under the stress of an epidemic, so too did attitudes toward religion. From the plague of Athens onwards, people either sought solace in religious practices or fled from Gods which had failed them (...). (3–4)

Beginning with the Greeks, these ideologies and perceptions of plague have continued to affect modern thinking on the subject of disease epidemics. It is precisely for this reason that Longrigg notes the impossibility of reading any writings produced during times of pestilence without first taking into consideration the classical accounts such as that of Thucydides.[4] Despite their various social, cultural, political and historical contexts, reactions to plague cannot help but resonate with these echoes from the past.

In the conclusion to his 1988 dissertation on the influence of plague and pestilence in Late Middle English texts, Edwin Stieve touched upon exactly what it is that unites both medical and literary plague writing of the past and the present. In his view, the greatest common denominator of plague writing is based on the idea of order.

> Medical writers explained that plague had come about as the result of distant and near causes, from the conjunction of planets and pestilential atmosphere. Moral writers, whose interpretation was rooted in the Bible and explained by the Church Fathers, stressed that human sin caused God to release plague on earth through natural forces. The difference between these two positions was not so much a difference between truth and error as it was an expression of the two traditional causes of plague: the spiritual forces of sin and the physical forces of nature. (...) Medical authorities had taught that plague imbalanced the humors and unless this balance was restored through phlebotomy or remedies, death would result. (...) The moral tradition taught that the body housed the soul; both should work harmoniously as part of a larger, divine plan. Writers who held a moral view believed that plague resulted from poor governance of both soul and body. (234–236)

As we have seen exemplified in the documents presented, where the purely medical writer tried to address the restoration of order at the physical level—such as through the regulation of diet and the correction of imbalances in the four humors—the literary writer shows a similar desire to move his intended audience towards a restoration of divine order. As noted, this can take the form of overtly didactic works that stress the perils of sin and the benefits of maintaining religious constancy. It is clear from historical documents written during the time of widespread plague outbreaks that it is this moral, rather than the expected physical, restoration of order that aroused the greatest level of interest among the writers of the time.

The idea that plague outbreaks resulted in a perceived disorder among of the physical forces of nature is a concept that is easy to understand from what we know of Medieval society. When faced with a lethal disease of epidemic proportions, the natural result would be a movement toward attempting to explain the onset of plague as a consequence of physical imbalances such as planetary anomalies or loss of equilibrium in one or more of the basic humors. However, it was the recognized disorder of plague contemporaries at the moral level that was harder to predict. While one would expect that medieval plague—a disease with an unknown pathology of vast magnitude—would have inspired greater piety among the survivors who viewed the visitation as a punishment from God, history has shown us that the direct result is actually one of moral disorder. This morbid disorder, which was also noted by Boccaccio, is explicitly detailed by plague chronicler, Matteo Villani:

> It was thought that the people, whom God by his grace had preserved in life, having seen the extermination of their neighbors and of all the nations of the world (...) would become better, humble, virtuous and catholic, avoiding iniquities and sins and overflowing with love and charity for one another. But (...) the opposite happened. Men, finding themselves few and rich by inheritances and successions of earthly things, forgetting the past as if it never was, gave themselves to the most disordered and sordid behavior than ever before. As they wallowed in idleness, their dissolution led them into the sin of gluttony, into banquets, taverns, delicate foods, and gambling. They rushed headlong into lust (...). And without any restraint almost all our city took up this shameful style of life; the other cities and provinces of the world did the same or worse. (*Cronica di Matteo Villani*, I, 10–11)

Accentuated by the rapid progression of plague throughout the cities, death came to be a source of revulsion. Consequently, revelry and moral disorder came to be a way of mounting a desperate rebellion against this biological process. The philosophy of "eat, drink, and be merry, for tomorrow we die" was taken to extremes in graveyard orgies that were common throughout Europe during the time of plague.[5] For example,

> At Avignon by the late fourteenth century, the cemetery of Champfleur had become, at least by repute, a place of debauchery. In 1393 a papal official threatened with excommunication those who dared "to dance, fight, throw iron or wooden bars, to play with wheels, to bowl, or play dice or other unseemly games or commit other unseemly acts' over the graves of the dead." Prostitutes solicited in cemeteries, and, by the testimony of contemporaries, fornicators and adulterers trysted among the graves. (Herlihy, 64)

In Spain, this idea of moral imbalance can even be connected to the reactionary slaughter of the Jews who were commonly blamed for disseminating the plague through the alleged poisoning of Christian wells.[6] Combining the unchallenged rule of vices with the failings of the clergy due to death or flight that we noted in chapter 3, the resulting moral disorder was an acute byproduct of plague. It was also the reason that contemporary writers of literature actively molded their work in an attempt to restore order through contrition and repentance. To them, the restoration of divine order and the aversion to plague went hand in hand.

This unifying idea of order and its relationship to all forms of Medieval plague writing—be they medical or literary in nature—are very closely related to the theories we have presented by the scholars Fass Leavy, Girard and Steele. First and foremost, each critic readily admits that there is a decided absence of literature, painting and sculpture that make a direct reference to the lethal epidemic that unquestionably raged near the moment of artistic production. However, each scholar in question also does not hesitate to affirm that the influence of plague on these forms of artistic expression is undeniably present regardless of any explicit reference. As Steel concludes, the epidemic's lethal and unpredictable nature in itself is what lends itself so readily to artistic representation.

> Because illness involves physical and emotional suffering it might be expected to cut more keenly than other aspects of life into the artist's sensibility. Living after all is most felt at the pitch of pleasure or at the height of pain which can be overlapping areas of feeling as the romantic understanding of love as a sickness well illustrates. However, whereas in life influenza is as common an occurence [sic] as love, in literature this is not the case. 'Flu seems somehow not to have seized the creative imagination. Still less has rheumatism. It would appear that in literature there is an order of attraction where illness is concerned. (...) The idea of plague seems to have been as powerful as the disease was virulent. More consistently than other illnesses it has seized the creative imagination of writers from the medieval period to the twentieth century. (88–89)

In fact, the perceived absence of any "real changes" that can be directly attributed to medieval plague actually has more to do with the mindset with which we approach works produced during virulent times than with these works themselves. We, as critics, tend to search all forms of plague literature for drastic changes or thematic innovations that mirror the intensity of the biological calamity itself. However, as history has repeatedly demonstrated, when humans are faced with cataclysmic disasters such as disease, famine or war, there is a greater tendency to look to previous forms of expression than to the innovation of new ones. It is only by returning to such previously established modes of thought—be it in medicine by adapting ideas of Galen or in literature by modeling Thucydides—would the plague writer be able to put a sense of order into what could easily be portrayed as disordered pestilential times.

Rather than looking for abrupt changes in writings produced near the times of pestilential epidemics, one should instead analyze these works for the subtle changes they make in the continuation of already established modes of expression for it is this continuation that leads to stability and, consequently, order. The relationship between disease and disorder has long been established by critics such as Susan Sontag. For example, in *Illness as Metaphor*, she makes the following connection:

> Order is the oldest concern of political philosophy, and if it is plausible to compare the polis to an organism, then it is plausible to compare civil disorder to an illness. The classical formulations which analogize a political disorder to an illness—from Plato to, say, Hobbes—presuppose the classical medical (and political) idea of balance. Illness comes from imbalance. Treatment is aimed at restoring the right balance—in political terms, the right hierarchy. The prognosis is always, in principal, optimistic. Society, by definition, never catches a fatal disease. (76)

Faced with both the physical and moral disorder that was the resulting byproduct of plague, writers of all types would naturally refer back to their literary antecedents in an attempt to explain—or cure as the case may be—that which they themselves did not understand. This is precisely why Stieve notes that, despite the unquestioned ferocity of the ravages of plague in Medieval England, contemporary chroniclers, medical and literary writers often referred to the disease in terms that were chronologically distant from their own.

> In Middle English literary works particularly, not only the warning of plague itself, but the catastrophic circumstances in which it occurred were derived from biblical commonplaces rather than from examples taken from the ravages of contemporary life. (239)

Polzer also notices these same absences of direct references to the plague that he believes unquestionably influenced the late medieval fascination with natural death and decay (107). In his study of early Italian frescoes, he notes:

> It is significant that the many texts and figures of the dead on our frescoes, as they can be discerned or as they have been transmitted by way of Renaissance copies, do not refer to the plague in any way. Its symptoms are quite obvious; the plague was substantially of the bubonic type, as we know from Boccaccio and other contemporary sources, causing dark swellings to develop at the neck, the armpit, the groin, sometimes as large as an egg or apple. The pneumonic plague which also raged involved coughing, a more common symptom. (...) Coeval illustrations of the Black Death have not been found, as far as I know, in Italian art. (...) Specific illustrations of the plague from the Renaissance are rare. (111)

Despite the fact that none of the dead portrayed in the frescoes bear the signs of plague, this critic concludes exactly what we are trying to suggest here. Namely, that the contemporary artist would have had a preference to established allegorical themes and medical precedents upon which to model their own work. In Polzer's opinion, it is basic human nature combined with common sense that provides the answers in support of this hypothesis.

Taking into account the documented reactions to plague that we have presented in this study, it is clear that the turmoil provoked by this disease took on various forms in Spain as well as in the rest of Europe.[7] Among the more conspicuous responses to this biological calamity were isolation and flight from the infected cities. It is precisely this response that leads Polzer to the conclusion that the Italian artists he refers to in his study would have had little time for the actual painting of frescoes during the plague due to the turbulence caused by the disease (119). In his view,

> The disruptive power of the great pandemic of 1348, destroying suddenly one-third to one-fourth of the population of western Europe, created conditions of chaos and social disruption so severe that they certainly terminated significant artistic production of any kind while the plague raged. Only retrospectively did man assess this extreme catastrophe in artistic and literary terms, as did Boccaccio in his *Decameron*. (...) As the plague returned periodically after the Black Death (...), a plague iconography gradually evolved reflecting the personal and collective yearning for protection. (126)

This iconography can be seen as a way in which humans try to come to term with the reality that surrounds him. Faced with an biological calamity of unknown origin, they would have certainly turned to the words of their predecessors—be they medical or literary in nature—for clues in trying to make sense of that which they could not comprehend. It is in the words of earlier authors that these later writers would have found some stability. "The accounts of the [plague] chroniclers are (...) abundant evidence of contemporary anguish over the Black Death," writes Nancy Siraisi, "yet existing modes of thought and expression provided ways of venting and coping with that anguish" (18). Far from reflecting the calamitous nature of plague through innovative forms of writing, both the medical and literary writers actually embraced the traditions established by their predecessors in an attempt to restore order through established frameworks. Despite the noted micro-changes we have outlined in the previous chapters, this movement toward a restoration of order is exactly what encapsulates what occurs in the various forms of plague writing in medieval Spain.

As I have commented in the introduction, this study is in no way a comprehensive summary of all forms of medical and literary writing produced near the times of pestilential outbreaks in Early Modern Spain. Rather, what I have attempted to do here is bring together for the first time a collection of works that, taken together, offer us valuable insight as to the nature of human reactions to plague at both the more scientific as well as at the purely imaginative levels. I have demonstrated that these seemingly independent forms of writing are connected not only to one another but also to historically distant episodes of disease and disease writing. Plague has been a powerful recurrent event that has affected both human experience and cultural imagination since classical antiquity and continues to do so until today. As a creative symbol, its pervasiveness in modern artistic works bears witness to this continuing influence and although outbreaks of this particular disease are quite rare today, there is no lack of popular substitutes. Grisly tales such as Pierre Ouellette's *The Third Pandemic* (Pocket Books, 1996), Stephen King's novel and 1990 movie, *The Stand* (Doubleday, 1978), and feature films such as *Outbreak* (1995), *Twelve Monkeys* (1995) and *The Rock* (1996) all demonstrate the continued popularity of themes based on microbiological disasters. When considered individually, none of these works allows for much insight as to the nature of human reaction to pandemic disease. However, when taken as a whole in the greater context of all forms of plague writing, the true significance of writing in a mortal world emerges.

Notes

1. Horrox, pp. 230–231.
2. As a reply to the comments of Verlinden, Shirk also recognizes the importance of the recurring plague epidemics that occurred subsequent to the Black Death: "As others have pointed out (especially Carpentier 1962b: 224–4 And Menéndez Pidal 1966: 482), the damages of the first plague were not irrepairable [sic]. It was the repetition of these effects in subsequent epidemics which caused irreversible harm" (366).
3. In a more recent review of Verlindin's conclusions about plague in the Iberian Peninsula, William D. Phillips, Jr. touches upon the more notable economic and political consequences of the disease. While affirming that Verlinden's conclusions can stand as supported by the limited scope of his investigations, Phillips readily acknowledges that both he as well as the vast majority of scholars have neglected the areas where plague certainly had the most impact: the cultural and psychological levels.

   > But he [Verlinden] left out, and so have I, attention to the psychological and cultural ramifications of the plague. Artistic and literary reactions to the Black Death were widespread, persistent, and influential in the century and a half after 1350. Abiding psychological and emotional reactions, as Iberians absorbed the horrible realities of the death toll and lived with the fear and insecurity that the plague engendered, shaped individual and collective actions in all fields. (62)

4. See "Epidemic, ideas and classical Athenian society," 27.
5. Steel also comments that more modern dramas also accentuate "the almost carnival spirit of desperate enjoyment that overcame certain sections of the population during plague epidemics" that was frequently noted by contemporary plague witnesses (95). See his article, *Plague Writing*, 93–96.
6. Rampant in especially in the North of Spain and the South of France in 1348 and 1349, the massacre of the Jews was so intense in certain cities that on July 5, 1348, Pope Clement VI was forced to reissue the bull *Sicut Judeis*—an order which essentially extended the Church's protection to the Jews. He would later follow up this document with subsequent affirmations of this order with the added theory that these false accusations are the direct result of immoral Christians who greedily sought to take possession of Jewish wealth. For translated

reproductions of actual documents commenting instances of well-poisoning by Jews in Spain, see Horrox, chapter V: Human Agency, 207–226.

7. George Deaux provides interesting commentary on the subject:

> Spain suffered as did the rest of Europe, not only from the ravages of the disease but from the demoralization and disorganization that followed it. Gilles Li Muisis includes in his account of the Black Death in Tournay a report of the pestilence in Spain he had received from a pilgrim to Compostella. The pilgrim and a companion, on their return, passed through Galicia and stopped for a night at a town he calls Salvaterra at the foot of the Pyrenees. The town, the pilgrim reported, was so hard hit by the plague that not one in ten of its people remained alive. (...) The Black Death's royal victims included Alfonso XI of Castile who died of plague while besieging Gibraltar in 1350. The Queen of Aragon, too, had been one of the earliest victims. But for the King, Peter IV, the Ceremonious, of Aragon, the Black Death worked some good to compensate for his loss. During a war with the unruly nobles of Aragon and Valencia, he was captured and held in Valencia; but the Black Death caused such havoc among his captors that he was able to escape, gather his forces and overthrow his enemies at the battle of Epila in July 1348. (114–115)

Bibliography

Primary Sources

Aragón, Sovereign 1336–1387 Peter IV. *Documentos Acerca De La Peste Negra En Los Dominios De La Corona De Aragón.* Ed. Amada López de Meneses. Zaragoza: Escuela de estudios medievales, 1956.

Chirino, Alonso de. *Menor Daño De La Medicina.* Ed. María Teresa Herrera. Salamanca: U de Salamanca, 1973.

Connolly, Jane E. *Translation and Poetization in the Quaderna Vía: Study and Edition of the 'Libro De Miseria D'Omne.'* Madison: The Hispanic Seminary of Hispanic Studies, 1987.

Ephesus, John of. *Joannis Episcopi Ephesi Syri Monophysitae Commentarii De Beatis Orientalibus Et Historiae Ecclesiasticae Fragmenta.* Trans. W. J. and J. P. N. Land Van Douwen. Amsterdam: Verhandelingen der Koninklijke Akademie van Nederland, 1889.

Infantes, Víctor. *Dança General De La Muerte.* Madrid: Visor, 1982.

Procopius of Caesarea. *History of the Wars I.* Trans. H.B. Dewing. London: William Heinemann, 1916.

Sánchez, María Nieves. *Tratados De La Peste.* Madrid: Arco Libros, 1993.

"Revelación De Un Hermitanno." *Biblioteca De Autores Españoles: Poetas Anteriores Al Siglo XV.* Ed. Tomás Antonio Sánchez. Vol. 57. Madrid: M. Rivadeneyra, 1864.

Scholasticus, Evagrius. "History of the Church by Theodoret and Evagrius." *Ecclesiastical History of Evagrius.* London: Henry G. Bohn, 1854.

Thucydides. *The Peloponnesian War.* Trans. Rex Warner. Middlesex: Penguin, 1954.

Secondary Sources

Ariès, Philippe. *Western Attitudes Toward Death: From the Middle ages to the Present.* Trans. Patricia M. Ranum. Baltimore: Johns Hopkins UP, 1974.

Allen, Pauline. *Evagrius Scholasticus the Church Historian.* Leuven: Spicilegium Sacrum

Lovaniense, 1981.

———. "The 'Justinianic' Plague." *Byzantion* 49 (1979): 5–20.

Amasuno, Marcelino V. *Contribución Al Estudio Del Fenómeno Epidémico En La Castilla De La Primera Mitad Del Siglo XV: El <<Regimiento Contra La Pestilencia>> De Alfonso López De Valladolid*. Valladolid: U de Valladolid, 1988.

———. "The Converso Physician in the Anti-Jewish Controversy in Fourteenth-Fifteenth Century Castile." *Medicine and Medical Ethics in Medieval and Early Modern Spain: an Intercultural Approach*. Eds. Samuel S. and Luís García-Ballester Kottek. Jerusalem: The Hebrew U, 1996. 92–118.

———. *Medicina Castellano-Leonesa Bajo Medieval*. Valladolid: Universidad de Valladolid, 1991.

———. "La Medicina y El Físico En La Danca General De La Muerte." *Hispanic Review* 1.65 (1997): 1–24.

Arrizabalaga, Jon. "Facing the Black Death: Perceptions and Reactions of University Medical Practitioners." *Practical Medicine From Salerno to the Black Death*. Eds. Luis García-Ballester. Cambridge: Cambridge UP, 1994. 237–88.

Benedictow, Ole J. *The Black Death (1346-1353): The Complete History*. Woodbridge: Boydell P, 2004.

Bennassar, Bartolomé. *Recherches Sur Les Grandes Épidémies Dans Le Nord De LEspagne à La Fin Du XIVe Siècle*. Paris: PU du Mirail, 1969.

Biraben, J. N. and Jacques Le Goff. "The Plague in the Early Middle Ages." *Biology of Man in History*. Eds. Robert Forster and Orest Ranum. Baltimore: Johns Hopkins UP, 1975. 48–80.

Boccaccio, Giovanni. *The Decameron*. Trans. G. H McWilliam. London: Penguin Books, 1972.

Boeckl, Christine M. *Images of Plague and Pestilence: Iconography and Iconology*. Kirksville: Truman State UP, 2000.

Bowsky, William M. *The Black Death: A Turning Point in History?* New York: Holt, Rinehart and Winston, 1971.

Bratton, Timothy L. "The Identity of the Plague of Justinian." *Transactions and Studies of the College of Physicians of Philadelphia* 3.2–3.3 (1981): 113–24; 174–180.

Bray, R. S. *Armies of Pestilence: The Impact of Disease on History*. New York: Barnes & Noble, 1996.

Calvi, Giulia. *Histories of a Plague Year: the Social and the Imaginary in Baroque Florence*. Trans. Dario Biocca and Bryant T. Ragan Jr. Berkeley: U of California P, 1984.

Cameron, Averil. *Procopius and the Sixth Century*. London: Gerald Duckworth and Company, 1985.

Campbell, Anna Montgomery. *The Black Death and Men of Learning*. 1931. New York: AMS Press, 1966.

Carmichael, Ann G. *Plague and the Poor in Renaissance Florence*. New York: Cambridge UP, 1986.

Carreras Panchón, Antonio. *La Peste y Los Médicos En La España Del Renacimiento.* Salamanca: Instituto de Historia de la Medicina Española, 1976.

———. "Aspectos médicos." *Cuadernos: Historia 16. La Peste Negra* 17 (1985): 6–11.

Cohn, Samuel K., Jr. *The Cult of Rembrance and the Black Death: Six Renaissance Cities in Central Italy.* Baltimore: Johns Hopkins UP, 1992.

Defoe, Daniel. *A Journal of the Plague Year.* Ed. Paula R. Backscheider. New York: Norton & Co., 1992.

Deyermond, Alan D. "El Ambiente Social e Intelectual De La *Danza De La Muerte.*" *Actas Del Tercer Congreso Internacional De Hispanistas.* México: El Colegio de México, 1970. 267–76.

———. *A Literary History of Spain: The Middle Ages.* London: Ernest Benn Limited, 1971.

Dohar, William J. *The Black Death and Pastoral Leadership: The Diocese of Hereford in the Fourteenth Century.* Philadelphia: U of Pennsylvania P, 1995.

Fass Leavy, Barbara. *To Blight With Plague: Studies in a Literary Theme.* New York: New York UP, 1992.

Felkel, Robert William. *The Theme of Desengaño in Spanish Dances of Death from the Fourteenth to the Seventeenth Century.* Diss. Michigan State U, 1973.

García-Ballester, Luis. "Changes in the *Regimina Sanitatis*: The Role of the Jewish Physicians." *Health, Disease and Healing in Medieval Culture.* Eds. Sheila Campbell et al. New York: St. Martin's Press, 1992. 119–31.

Girard, René. "The Plague in Literature and Myth." *Theories of Myth: From Ancient Israel and Greece to Freud, Jung, Campbell, and Lévi-Strauss.* Ed. Robert A. Segal. New York: Garland, 1996. 155–72.

Gottfried, Robert S. *The Black Death.* New York: The Free Press, 1983.

Gregg, Charles T. *Plague! The Shocking Story of a Dread Disease in America Today.* New York: Charles Scribner's Sons, 1978.

Guthke, Karl S. *The Gender of Death: A Cultural History in Art and Literature.* Cambridge: Cambridge UP, 1999.

Gyug, Richard Francis. *The Diocese of Barcelona During the Black Death.* Toronto: Pontifical Institute of Medieval Studies, 1994.

———. "The Effects and Extent of the Black Death of 1348: New Evidence for Clerical Mortality in Barcelona." *Mediaeval Studies* 45 (1983): 385–98.

Hamilton, Earl J. *Money, Prices, and Wages in Valencia, Aragon, and Navarre, 1351–1500.* Cambridge: Harvard UP, 1936.

Hecker, J. F. C. *The Epidemics of the Middle Ages.* Translator B. G. Babington. London: George Woodfall and Son, 1846.

Herlihy, David. *The Black Death and the Transformation of the West.* Cambridge: Harvard UP, 1997.

Hillgarth, J. N. *The Spanish Kingdoms: 1250–1516* Vol. II. Oxford: Clarendon P, 1978.

Hirst, L. Fabian. *The Conquest of Plague*. Oxford: Clarendon, 1953.

Horrox, Rosemary. *The Black Death*. Manchester: Manchester UP, 1994.

Huizinga, Johan. *The Waning of the Middle Ages*. New York: Doubleday, 1954.

Jillings, Karen. *Scotland's Black Death: The Foul Death of the English*. Stroud: Tempus, 2003.

Kelly, Maria. *The Great Dying: The Black Death in Dublin*. Stroud: Tempus, 2003.

Ladner, Gerhart B. "Medieval and Modern Understanding of Symbolism: a Comparison." *Speculum: a Journal of Medieval Studies* (1979): 223–56.

Lerner, Robert E. "The Black Death and Western European Eschatological Mentalities." *The Black Death: The Impact of the Fourteenth-Century Plague*. Ed. Daniel Williman. Binghamton: Center for Medieval and Early Renaissance Studies, 1982. 77–105.

Longrigg, James. "Epidemic, Ideas and Classical Athenian Society." *Epidemics and Ideas: Essays on the Historical Perception of Pestilence*. Eds. Terence Ranger and Paul Slack. Cambridge: Cambridge UP, 1992. 21–44.

López de Menses, Amada. *Documentos Acerca De La Peste Negra En Los Dominios De La Corona De Aragón*. Estudios De La Edad Media De La Corona De Aragón VI, páginas 291 a 447. Zaragoza: Consejo superior de investigaciones científicas, 1956.

McNeill, William H. *Plagues and Peoples*. New York: Doubleday, 1976.

McVaugh, Michael R. *Medicine Before the Plague: Practitioners and Their Patients in the Crown of Aragon, 1285–1345*. Cambridge: Cambridge UP, 1993.

Meiss, Millard. *Painting in Florence and Sienna After the Black Death*. 1951. Princeton: Princeton UP, 1978.

Mitre Fernández, Emilio. "La epidemia arrasa Europa." *Cuadernos: Historia 16. La Peste Negra* 17 (1985): 12–18.

Olson, Glending. *Literature as Recreation in the Later Middle Ages*. Ithaca: Cornell UP, 1983

Phillips, William D Jr. "*Peste Negra*: The Fourteenth-Century Plague Epidemics in Iberia." *On the Social Origins of Medieval Institutions: Essays in Honor of Joseph F. O'Callaghan*. Eds. Donald J. Kagay and Theresa M. Vann. Vol. 19. Boston: Brill, 1998. 47–62.

Platt, Colin. *King Death: the Black Death and Its Aftermath in Late-Medieval England*. Toronto: U of Toronto P, 1996.

Poe, Edgar Allan. *The Complete Tales and Poems of Edgar Allan Poe*. New York: Barnes and Noble, 1992.

Polzer, Joseph. "Aspects of Fourteenth-Century Iconography of Death and the Plague." *The Black Death: The Impact of the Fourteenth-Century Plague*. Ed. Daniel Williman. Binghamton: Center for Medieval and Early Renaissance Studies, 1982.

Rail, Chester David. *Plague Ecotoxicology*. Springfield: Charles C. Thomas, 1985.

Rather, L. J. "The "Six Things Non-Natural": A Note on the Origins and Fate of a Doctrine and a Phrase." *Clio Medica* 3 (1968): 337–47.

———. "Systematic Medical Treatises From the Ninth to the Nineteenth Century: The Unchanging Scope and Structure of Academic Medicine in the West." *Clio Medica* 11.4 (1976): 289–305.

Renouard, Yves. "The Black Death As a Major Event in World History." *The Black Death: A Turning Point in History?* Editor William M. Bowsky. Davis: Holt, Rinehard and Winston, 1971. 25–34.

Russell, Josiah C. "That Earlier Plague." *Demography* 5.1 (1968): 174–84.

Shirk, Melanie V. "The Black Death in Aragon, 1348–1351." *Journal of Medieval History* 7 (1981): 357–67.

Sobrequés Callicó, Jaime. "La Peste Negra En La Península Ibérica." *Anuario De Estudios Medievales* VII (1973): 67–102.

Steel, David. "Plague Writing: From Boccaccio to Camus." *Journal of European Studies* 11.2 (1981): 88–110.

Stieve, Edwin M. *Medical and Moral Interpretations of Plague and Pestilence in Late Middle English Texts.* Diss. Michigan State U, 1988.

Tristram, Philippa. *Figures of Life and Death in Middle English Literature.* New York: New York UP, 1976.

Twigg, Graham. *The Black Death: a Biological Reappraisal.* London: Batsford Academic and Educational, 1984.

Valdeón, Julio. "La Muerte Negra En La Península." *Cuadernos: Historia 16. La Peste Negra* 17 (1985): 19–27.

Verlinden, Charles. "Spain: A Temporary Setback." *The Black Death: A Turning Point in History?* Editor William M. Bowsky. Davis: Holt, Rinehart and Winston, 1971.

Viña Liste, José María. *Cronología De La Literatura Española: I) Edad Media.* Madrid: Cátedra, 1991.

Whyte, Florence. *The Dance of Death in Spain and Catalonia.* Baltimore: Waverly P, 1931.

Ziegler, Philip. *The Black Death.* 1969. Wolfeboro Falls: Alan Sutton Publishing, 1991.

Studies in the Humanities

Edited by Guy Mermier

The Studies in the Humanities series welcomes manuscripts discussing various aspects of the humanities. The series' emphasis is on medieval and Renaissance literatures with a focus on Western civilizations and cultures. Submissions dealing with linguistics, history, politics, or sociology within the same time frame and geographical bounds are also encouraged. Manuscripts may be submitted in English, French, or Italian. The preferred style manual is the MLA Handbook (1995).

For additional information about this series or for the submission of manuscripts, please contact:

>Dr. Heidi Burns
>Peter Lang Publishing, Inc.
>P.O. Box 1246
>Bel Air, MD 21014-1246

To order other books in this series, please contact our Customer Service Department:

>(800) 770-LANG (within the U.S.)
>(212) 647-7706 (outside the U.S.)
>(212) 647-7707 FAX

or browse online by series:

>WWW.PETERLANG.COM